SPORTS INJURY MANAGEMENT
A Quarterly Series

EVALUATION OF
Isokinetic
Equipment

VOLUME 1, NUMBER 1, MARCH 1988

SPORTS INJURY MANAGEMENT
A Quarterly Series

EVALUATION OF
Isokinetic
Equipment

VOLUME 1, NUMBER 1, MARCH 1988

TERRY R. MALONE, Ed.D., P.T., A.T.C.

Series Editor
Executive Director of Sports Medicine
Associate Professor of Physical Therapy
Assistant Professor of Surgery
Duke University
Durham, North Carolina

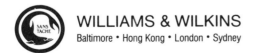
WILLIAMS & WILKINS
Baltimore • Hong Kong • London • Sydney

Editor: John P. Butler
Managing Editor: Linda Napora
Design: Norman W. Och
Illustration Planning: Lorraine Wrzosek
Production: Anne G. Seitz

88 89 90 91 92
1 2 3 4 5 6 7 8 9 10

SERIES EDITOR'S FOREWORD

Sports injury management (SIM) has been designed for the clinician practicing in sports medicine environments. It is specifically geared to sports physical therapists and athletic trainers wishing to stay abreast of the constantly changing field of sports medicine.

Each volume (four issues) will cover clinical science, a regional anatomy problem, a specific sports injury, and a special topic. This format has been chosen to enable us to provide you with the current information you need.

Our plan for the first and second years follows:

1988

Special Topic—Evaluation of Isokinetic Equipment
Clinical Science—Muscle Injury and Rehabilitation
Regional Anatomy—Shoulder Injuries
Sports Injury—Basketball: Injuries and Treatment

1989

Special Topic—Thermal and Electrical Modalities
Clinical Science—Soft Tissue Mobilization
Regional Anatomy—Hand and Wrist Injuries and Treatment
Sports Injury—Soccer: Injuries and Treatment

We will be flexible and responsive. Reader comments/suggestions are welcomed and appreciated.

Terry R. Malone

PREFACE

Isokinetic exercise has become one of the most utilized modes of exercise. With this popularity has come an increase in the types of equipment available to control such movements. As the number of devices has increased, the difficulty with clinician assessment of equipment has increased as well. This volume has been designed to serve as a guide to computer-controlled/enhanced isokinetic equipment.

I would like to thank all of the clinicians who contributed and especially those who authored individual chapters dealing with specific pieces of equipment. Each of these individuals was given the opportunity to structure the chapter in the manner most efficacious for providing information on the utilization of that particular unit. Chapters were contributed by Cathy E. Busby (Ariel), Julie M. Chandler (Kin-Com), Anthony Delitto (Lido), D. Keith Kleven (MERAC), Thomas J. Sansone (Cybex), and Michael L. Voight (Biodex).

Terry R. Malone
Series Editor

CONTRIBUTORS

Kathy E. Busby, M.S., P.T.
Director
Capital Physical Therapy, Inc.
Raleigh, North Carolina

Julie M. Chandler, M.S., P.T.
Clinical Associate
Department of Physical Therapy
Duke University
Durham, North Carolina

Anthony Delitto, M.H.S., P.T.
Instructor, Program in Physical Therapy
Washington University School of Medicine
St. Louis, Missouri

D. Keith Kleven, M.S., P.T., A.T.C.
Director, Las Vegas Institute of
Physical Therapy and Sports Medicine
Las Vegas, Nevada

Thomas J. Sansone, M.A., P.T.
Physical Therapy
Islip, New York

Michael L. Voight, M.Ed., P.T., A.T.C.
Instructor, Division of Physical Therapy
University of Miami
Miami, Florida

CONTENTS

1

Introduction

Mechanically controlled isokinetic exercise was made available with the introduction of the Cybex I in the late 1960s. Clinicians have found this form of exercise to be extremely safe and efficacious in treating patients with a variety of musculoskeletal problems. Mechanical evaluation of muscular output via isokinetic exercise is possible through several devices. In this issue the clinician is provided with complete information on six products with isokinetic measurement capabilities.

The information was "compiled" from a variety of sources. Senior clinicians familiar with the "clinical" applications of each device agreed to share their expertise concerning this topic. The manufacturers provided technical assistance and photographs. Feedback regarding the advantages and disadvantages was requested from many users throughout the country.

Although clinicians must be able to evaluate muscular output in an objective fashion, it is important to determine what is required by their setting prior to the selection of testing equipment. The manufacturers of isokinetic devices provide a variety of options much like those confronting the customer attempting to purchase an automobile.

The material presented here will assist the clinician evaluating isokinetic equipment. It is recommended that clinicians visit others who are using multiple devices (more than one manufacturer) to "see" and "hear" their comments and those of their patients.

System specifications of the six devices discussed in this volume have a wide range. The basic skeletal specifications are presented below.

Systems Specifications

Ariel Computerized Exercise System (CES)

Manufacturer—
ARIEL DYNAMICS
22000 Plano Trabuco Road
Trabuco Canyon, CA 92678
(Distributed by Wilson Sporting
Goods)

Type of System—Passive

Controlling Methodology—Computer-controlled via hydraulic valve

Operational Modes—Isometric contractions, isokinetic contractions, concentric (variable resistance advertised as isotonic)

Speeds—0 to 1000 degrees/second (stated by manufacturer; not documented by a published work)

Torque—1000 ft-lb maximum (stated by manufacturer; not documented by published work)

Mechanical Stops—Yes, computer established

Accessories—Back/trunk testing accessory is available

Other Accessories—Available according to the manufacturer from other sources

Space Required—80 sq ft

Biodex System

Manufacturer—
Biodex Corporation
PO Box S
Shirley, NY 11967

Type of System—Active

Controlling Methodology—Servomotor via different systems according to operational mode (microprocessor)

Operational Modes—Passive motion, isokinetic exercise (concentric and eccentric contractions), isometrics

Speeds—30 to 450 degrees/second concentric
10 to 120 degrees/second eccentric

Torque—Maximum of 650 ft-lb concentric
Maximum of 150 ft-lb eccentric

Ramping—Yes, predetermined according to terminal velocity

Mechanical Stops—Variable

Computer Enhancement—IBM compatible

Accessories—Accessory chair for specific patterns; back/trunk accessory for flexion and extension

Space Required—64 to 80 sq ft; recommended: a minimum of 10 × 10 sq ft

Cybex
(340 System)

Manufacturer—
CYBEX
2100 Smithtown Ave
Ronkonkoma, NY 11779-0903

Type of System—Passive

Controlling Methodology—Electronic servomotor

Operational Modes—Isometric contraction and isokinetic (concentric)

Speeds—0 to 300 degrees/second

Torque—Maximum of 360 ft-lb

Ramping—Yes, adjustable

Computer Enhancement—Yes, IBM compatible

Accessories—Upper body testing table; accessory cart (back system is a separate unit)

Space Required—80 to 90 sq ft; recommended: 10 × 12 sq ft

Kin-Com System

Manufacturer—
Chattecx Corporation
PO Box 4287
Chattanooga, TN 37405

Type of System—Active

Controlling Methodology—Computer-controlled hydraulic servomechanism

Operational Modes—Passive motion, isokinetic (concentric and eccentric contractions), isometric

Speeds—0 to 210 degrees/second

Torque/Force—2200 Newtons maximum force (greater than 500 ft-lb)

Ramping—Yes, adjustable

Mechanical Stops—Yes (computer established)

Computer Enhancement—IBM (hard drive)

Accessories—Accessory chair for specific joint stabilization; back/trunk for flexion extension; EMG for specific correlative test involving contraction and documentation

Space Required—88 sq ft; recommended: 10 × 12 sq ft

Lido System

Manufacturer—
Loredan Biomedical
1632 DaVinci Court
Davis, CA 95616

Type of System—Both active and passive systems are available

Controlling Methodology—Computer-controlled hydraulic servovalve (passive system); computer-controlled servomotor (active system)

Operational Modes—Passive system is concentric, isokinetic; active system is isometric, isokinetic (concentric and eccentric), passive motion

Speeds—60 to 400 degrees/second concentric (passive system); 0 to 220 degrees/second eccentric limitations

Torque—400 ft-lb concentric maximum 250 ft-lb eccentric maximum (eccentric maximum is based on concentric movement but absolute maximum available through the unit is 250 ft-lb)

Mechanical Stops—Yes, computer established

Computer Enhancement—IBM-compatible system controls and provides enhancement of data

Accessories—Back system is separate, no specific accessories

Space Required—80 sq ft; recommended: 10 × 10 sq ft

MERAC System

Manufacturer—
Universal Gym Equipment
PO Box 127
930 27th Ave, SW
Cedar Rapids, IA 52406

Type of System—Passive

Controlling Methodology—Computer controlled via feedback loop, dedicated system

Operational Modes—Isometric, isotonic, isokinetic (concentric only), dynamic variable resistance

Speeds—500 degrees/second isokinetic

Torque—500 ft-lb maximum

Mechanical Stops—Yes, computer established

Accessories—Accessory chair for specific joint patterns; back/trunk flexion-extension accessory table available

Space Required—80 sq ft; recommended: 10 × 10 sq ft

2

Ariel Computerized Exercise System

The Ariel Computerized Exercise System (CES) is an advanced system that automatically monitors, controls, and modifies resistance and velocity while the user is exercising. It is a computerized hydraulic system and is superior to many hydraulic systems in that it is not limited by a fixed flow rate through the valve. The CES has a stored program computer which controls a feedback loop to the exercise mechanism; the valve that controls the flow of hydraulic fluid (which determines velocity and force) is automatically adjusted during exercise. Therefore, the CES is able to maintain desired patterns of force and is able to respond to an individual's performance. Thus the manufacturer calls it the "intelligent system" (1). Measurements within the hydraulic system are made by utilization of transducers for force, bar position, and velocity.

The design of this system makes maximal use of the microcomputer. Not only does it control the hydraulic resistance mechanism, it performs data measurement and display as well as system control. The system control console also controls two diskette drives to store and access data, and it controls specialized electronics that monitor and control each exercise station.

With the two diskette drives, a user may operate the CES in the programmed mode. In this mode, a preprogrammed diskette is inserted. Once a key is pressed to select the appropriate stored program, the user simply follows the on-screen instructions as the computer sets up each exercise (resistance, repetitions, rest time, etc.). When the session is complete at that station, the computer prompts the user to move to the next station or informs the user that the session is completed. Results are measured and saved automatically. More advanced operators can make use of the advanced feature, which enables programming individual exercise sequences designed to achieve specific results.

A color monitor displays information. During exercise it continuously displays performance graphically and numerically (Fig. 2.1). The monitor also displays the cumulative performance at the end of each exercise. After each exercise, the operator may choose to review any one of nine exercise results displays by pressing a single key. Results can be copied by a printer or stored on a diskette. Additional tabular and graphic results such as a comparison of data from several exercise sessions and left-

5

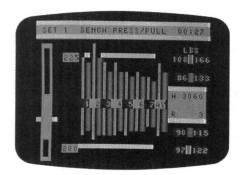

Figure 2.1. Display during exercise provides information about force, work, repetitions, and elapsed time.

right comparisons may be printed or saved. A printer buffer allows the exerciser to continue while results are being printed.

The desired exercise results to be viewed or printed are selected from a results menu (Fig. 2.2). A brief description of commonly saved results follows. The average curve plot (Fig. 2.3) is a graphic display of force through the range of motion. This curve is an average for all repetitions in the set of exercise. Results of three separate exercise sessions can be displayed for comparison. Rehabilitation curves (Fig. 2.4), commonly known as force curves, are a graphic display of force plotted against time for each individual repetition. Range of motion plotted against time is also displayed.

Rehabilitation statistics (Fig. 2.5) are a statistical analysis of various parameters of movement. Results of the up and down motion of the exercise are listed separately along with RMS (a statistical measure of variance from the average). A few of the more commonly used statistical measurements will be briefly explained. PK VAL and AVG VAL are the peak and average exercise values (either force or velocity). PK PWR and AVG PWR are the peak and average power values. POS(PK) is the point in the range of motion where peak force or velocity occurred. PK HOLD is the amount of time peak force or velocity was held. RECIP is the amount of time it takes for the user to reciprocate motion, i.e., to change from the up to the down direction.

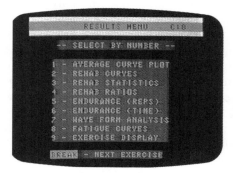

Figure 2.2. Exercise results are reported in nine different formats.

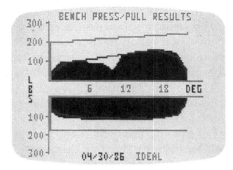

Figure 2.3. Average curve plot graphically illustrates average force through range of motion and can optionally compare values with previous performance.

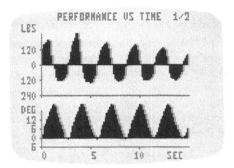

Figure 2.4. Rehabilitation curves demonstrate the measured force value and bar position for each exercise repetition.

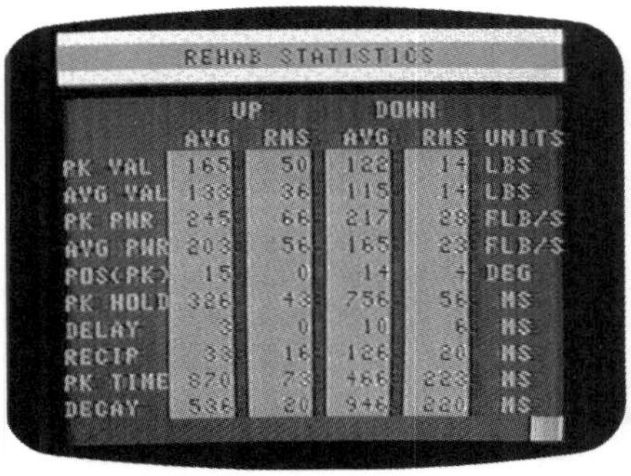

Figure 2.5. Various parameters of exercise performance are listed in the rehabilitation statistics report.

Rehabilitation ratios (Fig. 2.6) contain additional statistical data expressed as ratios. These include WORK, which is the quantity of work performed during exercise; work is reported separately for the up and down motions. UP/DN MAX and UP/DN AVG are the ratios of up to down measured exercise values expressed as percents. These allow a comparison of agonists to antagonists for maximum force as well as average force (2).

The complete CES consists of two exercise stations (Figs. 2.7 and 2.8). The multifunction exercise station (MES) and the arm, leg, back exercise station (AES) each allow a wide variety of exercise positions. Each station consists of a moveable exercise bar and an adjustable seat with stabilization straps. Because the exercise bar provides resistance by a computerized hydraulic mechanism, the design automatically adapts to individuals of different sizes and strength levels, eliminating the need for manual adjustment of the machine (1). The resistance on the bar can be set to be either unidirectional or bidirectional, and either unilateral or bilateral.

Special Features

1. The Ariel CES is not limited to one exercise mode. The microcomputer control of hydraulics allows this flexibility. Exercise modes include variable velocity (isokinetic), variable resistance (isotonic), and isometric.

2. The variable velocity and variable resistance modes are controllable throughout the range of motion. Velocity and force can be increased or decreased through the range, allowing acceleration. The increase or decrease can be linear, exponential, or programmed by the operator to achieve a curve of any shape. Isometric contractions can also be programmed to occur at any point in the range of motion.

3. The use of hydraulics allows safe, quiet exercise and overcomes the problem of inertia. Thus, a greater force is not necessary to begin an exercise and the bar does not tend to keep moving at the end. The design assures that the bar stops when released (3).

4. Microcomputer control of exercise allows a diskette to be created with either standard exercise programs or customized individual exercise sequences. This makes

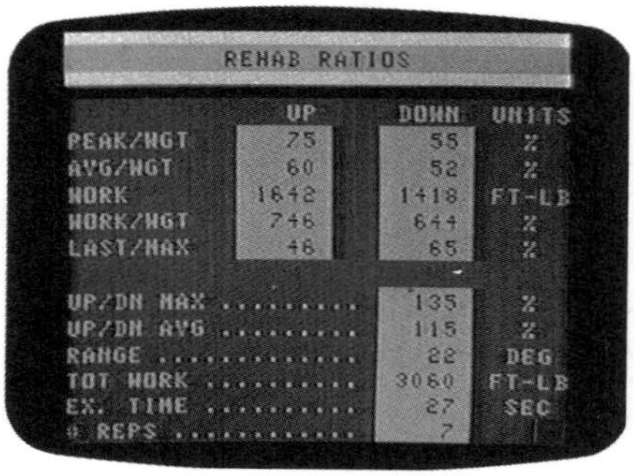

Figure 2.6. Rehabilitation ratios report is a listing of exercise performance values expressed as ratios.

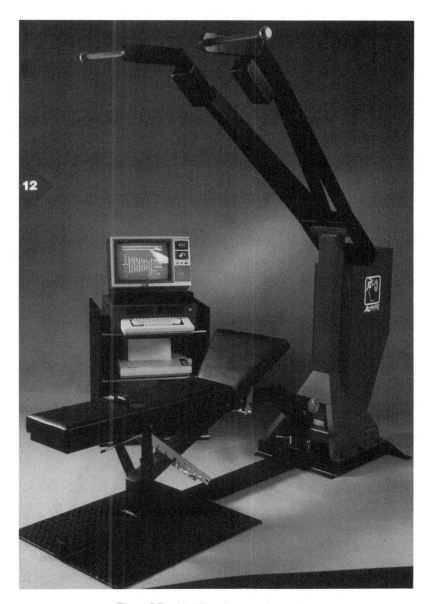

Figure 2.7. Multifunction exercise station.

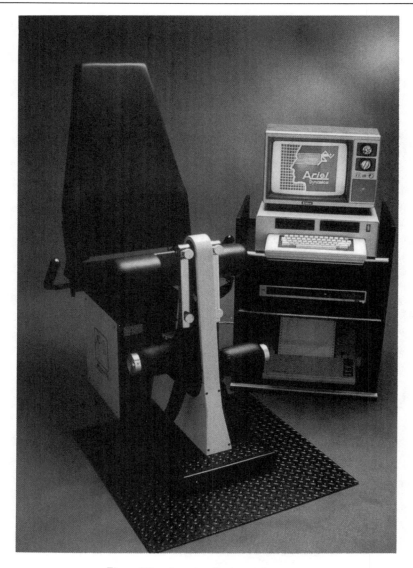

Figure 2.8. Arm, leg, back exercise station.

for ease of use by the physical therapist and allows the user to be as independent as possible. Set up time for each exercise is minimal.

5. The microcomputer and the sophisticated software allow the user to save, compute, print, and compare results data. The operator never needs to spend time calculating results and may view or print results after the user has completed the session.

6. Visual displays and audible tones give excellent feedback to the user and the physical therapist during and after exercise. A strong motivator is the ability to com-

pare current and previous performance data in color graphic form on the monitor after each exercise (Fig. 2.9). The operator may also preprogram target values which appear on the screen as the user is exercising.

7. A "pyramid" option allows the force or velocity to change from repetition to repetition within a set. Thus, the operator may program an exercise to get progressively easier or more difficult as the user exercises.

8. The "automatic" option changes force or velocity in a permanent manner from session to session. The operator may increase or decrease repetitions, quantity of work, percent fatigue, or exercise time from session to session.

Reliability and Validity

The manufacturer has provided abstracts of two separate studies of reliability and validity of the Ariel CES. The first study, done by the Department of National Defense in Canada (4), studied force measurement and angular velocity. Force measurement was examined by comparing the CES readout of an applied force to known calibration weights applied to the CES. Angular velocity was examined by comparing various velocities selected through software commands to the actual velocity measured with a microswitch activated timer. Intrasubject reproducibility was also studied. Their conclusion was that force measurements and angular velocities are valid and reproducible with the CES if the system is calibrated daily according to manufacturer's specifications (4).

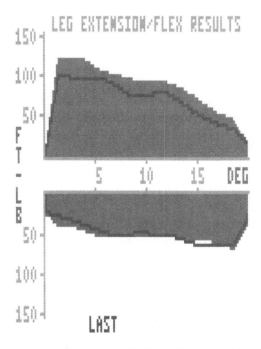

Figure 2.9. Average force curve for leg extension/flexion (solid graph) with a comparison to a previous session (line).

A second study of reproducibility was performed at Hahnemann University Hospital (5). In this study, 14 subjects performed several trials to assess the reproducibility of peak force, peak power, and total work. Speeds of 15 degrees/second and 100 degrees/second were selected. It was concluded that the selected strength parameters at the selected speeds are highly reproducible using the CES.

It appears that the CES, as utilized by the above groups, provided valid and reproducible data for the selected parameters at the speeds selected. More comprehensive studies with better design are necessary in order to conclude that data over a wide spectrum of velocities and for all strength parameters are valid and reliable. The manufacturer states maximum force measurable is 1000 pounds and maximum speed is 1000 degrees/second. Reliability and validity at these levels need to be established.

Multifunction Exercise Station (MES)

The MES design is similar to many traditional weight lifting stations. For athletes and other individuals with experience utilizing other weight equipment, the MES is easily adapted to, and it has excellent carry over value. At discharge from rehabilitation or to supplement the rehabilitation process, other weight equipment may be utilized more safely as individuals are familiar with their abilities in these traditional positions.

Another advantage to the design of this station is the ability to perform traditional strengthening exercises as well as many functional activities such as pushing, pulling, lifting, and squatting. It is well known that training is specific to position and activity. Because our goals are generally to return our patients to particular functional activities, we must often try to reproduce the activity as closely as possible in the clinic for maximum benefit. This is not generally feasible with exercise equipment which is designed primarily to isolate single-joint movement.

Some exercises that are possible with the MES are: bench press (Fig. 2.10); incline press (Fig. 2.11); overhead press (Fig. 2.12); squat (Fig. 2.13); arm curl (Fig. 2.14); abdominal curls (Fig. 2.15); and lifts (from midcalf to overhead) (Figs. 2.16 and 2.17). All exercises can be performed unidirectionally or bidirectionally and either unilaterally or bilaterally.

Clinical Utilization

An athlete being rehabilitated for a shoulder injury will be thoroughly tested initially. A testing diskette will store data such as force, power, force curves, range of motion, total work, and right versus left performance. An exercise diskette will be set up with either an individualized program or a previously established protocol. This diskette may contain several types of exercises such as bench press and incline press at several different angles. The program will indicate the desired range of motion, sets, repetitions, and rest periods, as well as exercise type (isotonic, isokinetic, etc.). When the athlete returns for rehabilitation, the user diskette is placed in the diskette drive and the program started. With proper instruction, the user can continue through all exercises with little supervision. As a motivational tool, the average force curve will be saved weekly for comparison. The user will then be able to compare his/her performance with that of the previous two weeks.

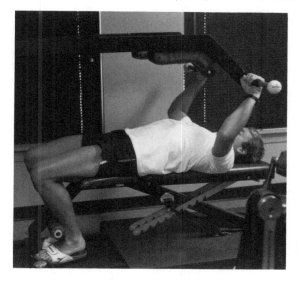

Figure 2.10. Bench press.

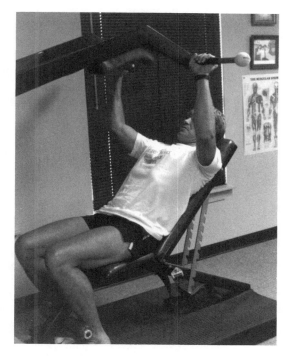

Figure 2.11. Incline press.

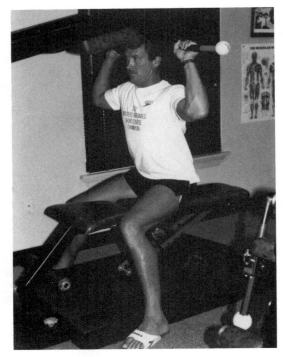

Figure 2.12. Overhead press.

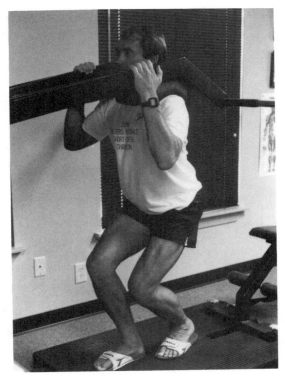

Figure 2.13. Squat.

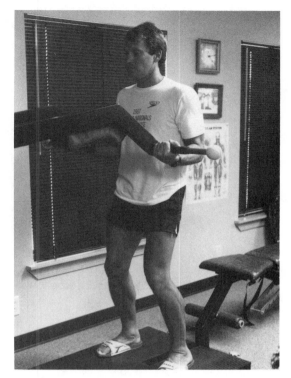

Figure 2.14. Arm curl.

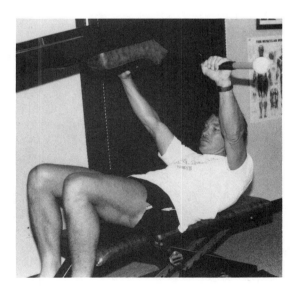

Figure 2.15. Abdominal curl (MES).

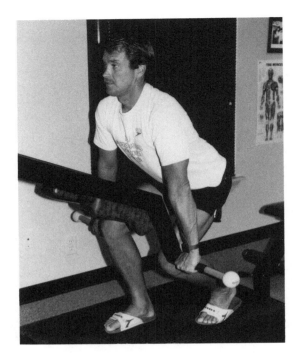

Figure 2.16. Lift: midcalf.

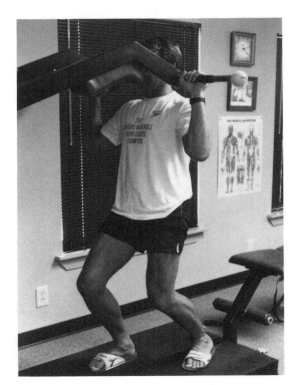

Figure 2.17. Lift: overhead.

When it is time to retest the user, the preprogrammed testing diskette is once again utilized. After completing the retest, reports can be generated with a variety of comparisons such as right to left (Fig. 2.18). This information is stored on the diskette and may be printed to be sent to physicians, trainers, etc.

Another use of the MES is for rehabilitation of back injuries. Once again, the user is tested initially, and desired information is stored on a diskette. Initial information may also be printed and sent to appropriate individuals. Often our patients with back injuries must return to work at jobs that involve repetitive lifting. Although strength is an important issue, the ability to sustain performance is often a more limiting factor. To build endurance, a diskette will be programmed for the user to perform a fixed amount of work. During rehabilitation, the user will perform several sets of a fixed amount of work in a particular lifting position. The diskette will be prepro-

```
          COTO RESEARCH CENTER
      PERFORMANCE PROGRESS 11/23/83
      USER: J.WISE
      EXERCISE: BENCH PRESS/PULL
      VALUES: 015/015  015/015 DG/S
      MODE: VEL    5 REPS
                  LEFT        RIGHT
               10/18  10/19  10/18  10/19  DATE
PK-FORCE   EX    44     38     49     44   LBS
           FL    46     46     44     44   LBS
           F/E  105    121     90    100   %
AV-FORCE   EX    35     30     41     35   LBS
           FL    38     38     35     33   LBS
           F/E  109    127     85     94   %
PK-POWER   EX    60     50     62     57   FLB/S
           FL    57     60     55     55   FLB/S
           F/E   95    120     89     96   %
AV-POWER   EX    40     36     50     45   FLB/S
           FL    45     45     43     40   FLB/S
           F/E  113    125     86     89   %
POS(PK)    EX    23     14     16     18   DEG
           FL    18     19     17     20   DEG
           F/E   78    136    106    111   %
PK HOLD    EX  1083    990   1066   1346   MS
           FL   860    966   1073    886   MS
           F/E   79     98    101     66   %
DELAY T    EX     3      3     10      3   MS
           FL    13     23     16     26   MS
           F/E  433    767    160    867   %
REC DLY    EX   276    256    250    160   MS
           FL   323    233    253    170   MS
           F/E  117     91    101     94   %
PK TIME    EX  1473   1013   1046   1233   MS
           FL   706    620    826    560   MS
           F/E   48     61     79     45   %
DECAY T    EX   606   1060   1073    706   MS
           FL  1360   1400   1353   1400   MS
           F/E  224    132    126    198   %
WORK       EX   418    371    506    421   FT-LB
           FL   464    469    464    389   FT-LB
           F/E  111    126     92     92   %
PK/WGT     EX    29     25     33     29   %
           FL    31     31     29     29   %
AV/WGT     EX    23     20     27     23   %
           FL    25     25     23     22   %
WORK/WGT   EX   279    247    337    261   %
           FL   309    313    309    259   %
TOT WORK        882    840    970    810   FT-LB
EX. TIME         23     22     23     21   SEC
RANGE            30     29     31     28   DEG
#REPS             5      5      5      5
```

Figure 2.18. Comparison results report for left vs. right bench press.

grammed to increase this amount of work by a set amount each session so that the workload becomes progressively more difficult.

The fatigue mode is another method of building endurance. The diskette is programmed such that exercise continues until two consecutive repetitions fall below a preset level. If 75% is the chosen value, the exercise set ends when the force of two repetitions goes below 75% of maximum.

Arm, Leg, Back Exercise Station (AES)

The AES allows more isolation of joint motion. The seat can be repositioned and the bar can be removed so that a variety of joints can be tested and exercised in various positions.

The AES can be utilized as it comes from the manufacturer for knee flexion-extension (Fig. 2.19), elbow flexion-extension (Fig. 2.20), abdominal curls, shoulder rotation, and pushing and pulling. An attachment can be purchased to test and exercise trunk flexion and extension (Fig. 2.21). This feature has not been utilized as yet by this clinic. It appears to be an attractive option, as it allows use of existing equipment rather than purchase of another piece of specialty equipment.

The exercise bar may be removed and other attachments added to allow isolated testing and exercise of virtually every major joint. However, no attachments are available from this manufacturer at this time. Attachments must be purchased from other manufacturers of isokinetic equipment. Positioning and stabilization of the patient are left to the imagination and ingenuity of the operator.

Clinical Utilization

A patient presenting with knee dysfunction may be tested isokinetically at a variety of speeds. By evaluating statistical data (Fig. 2.22), strength, power, and workload

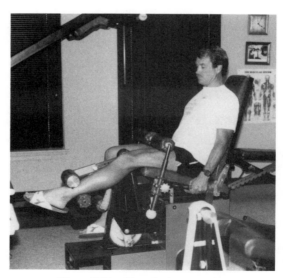

Figure 2.19. Knee flexion-extension.

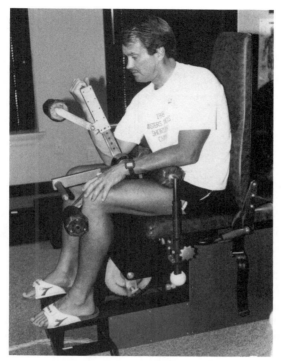

Figure 2.20. Elbow flexion-extension.

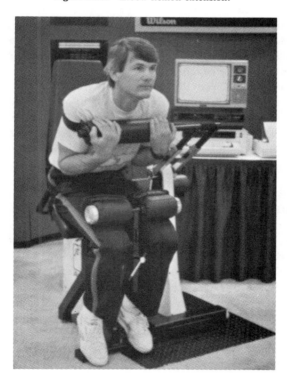

Figure 2.21. Back attachment to test and rehabilitate trunk flexion-extension.

Table Summary of Data (Up/Down)

Bar (Degrees)	Today (Ft-lb)	Bar (Degrees)	Today (Ft-lb)
0	12/18	32	51/41
4	86/29	36	36/42
8	97/30	40	28/44
12	93/30	44	27/45
16	79/37	48	30/46
20	72/39	52	39/47
24	64/39	56	48/45
28	60/39	60	51/44

Figure 2.22. Tabular results of an average force curve listing force values every 4 degrees.

deficits can be noted. The force curve for the involved knee may demonstrate a sudden abnormal drop in force output at a particular point in the range of motion. A tabular printout of force output every several degrees throughout the range of motion indicates exactly where the drop in force output occurred (Fig. 2.22). In programming the user diskette for rehabilitation, the operator can utilize this information to the maximal benefit of the user.

The operator will set up a program to exercise the user at a variety of speeds isokinetically. To strengthen the knee extensors at their weak point in the range of motion, the diskette can be programmed for a slower speed at that point in the range of motion or an isometric contraction for up to 6 seconds (allowing more time for recruitment). This has been a very effective mode of operation for improving strength at specific points in the range of motion.

The ability to monitor easily the total quantity of work and the average force through the range of motion have proven invaluable in our use of the CES. Average force through the range of motion may be a more important functional measure than peak force. In the case of knee testing and rehabilitation, peak force of the involved knee often equals the involved knee while there is still a deficit in total work and average force. Rehabilitation is not considered complete until these important measures are equal.

A common use of the variable velocity mode of operation in our clinic is exercise involving acceleration through the range of motion. Strictly isokinetic exercisers are limited to fixed velocity. An exercise such as knee extension may begin at 60 degrees/second and progress linearly to 220 degrees/second as the knee approaches full extension. This seems to simulate more closely the functional use of the extremity.

In testing and rehabilitation, it is sometimes preferable to set resistance, allowing traditional "weight lifting" exercise. The exercise diskette is programmed in the variable velocity mode. Resistance level may be set to any weight by merely pressing a key rather than by manually adding weights to a bar. Further, this weight can be increased or decreased on each repetition without interruption. This is a particularly valuable option for directing exercise programs that will be performed on the weight lifting equipment found in most nonclinical settings.

Advantages and Disadvantages

Advantages

1. Maximal use of the microcomputer to control exercise as well as compute data. The feedback loop allows safe, always maximal resistance. The computer does all calculations and comparisons. Only initially, must the operator spend time setting up the exercise program. The operator is also freed from calculating comparisons and ratios.

2. Flexibility of having many exercise modes in the same system (variable velocity, variable resistance, isokinetics, isotonics, and isometrics).

3. Versatility of the exercise stations. This allows functional movements as well as isolated joint movements with little set-up time. Two exercise stations allow two users to use the equipment simultaneously.

4. Ease of use. Little supervision of the user is necessary.

5. Feedback to the patient and operator during and after exercise.

6. Ability to store data for comparison and printout at a later time.

7. Accessibility to Dr. Gideon Ariel, developer of this exercise system. The opportunity to consult with the developer assists in maximal utilization of this system. The manufacturer also is receptive to suggestions and some changes have been made in response to suggestions from the field.

Disadvantages

1. This manufacturer does not make accessories to allow isolated movements of all joints; however, a selling feature is the fact that the bar is removable and other accessories can be added. These accessories were difficult to obtain from another manufacturer.

2. The equipment has undergone several changes since it was initially manufactured. At times this makes it difficult to get parts as components have changed. Further, not all new components are compatible with old components as the manufacturer indicated (however, in their defense, they have worked out excellent trade-in deals to upgrade the system).

3. The early models use Radio Shack color computers and CGP115 color graphic printers. The rationale was ease of service. These components are no longer available. We bought a spare used color computer and replaced the obsolete printers. Printer options do allow the use of other printers such as the Epson.

4. The later models have upgraded electronics and disc drives. The software package has also been upgraded for ease of operation.

5. They do not have local service but are very helpful on the phone. Someone on your staff with electronic or computer knowledge can be a great help.

Case Study

A 41-year-old man, a National Master's Champion Swimmer, presented with bilateral shoulder pain, greater on the right than left. He reported experiencing pain for approximately 2 years; the pain had worsened recently. Pain was only present while he was swimming, and it had been affecting his training. He had recently competed in the National Master's Championships and was beginning his off-season.

On evaluation, he was noted to have laxity of the anterior shoulder bilaterally. Manual muscle testing identified weakness in external rotation.

He was then tested in variable velocity mode on the Ariel CES in shoulder rotation. He was seated with the shoulder in 90 degrees of flexion for the initial testing (the standard protocol we utilize). Warm-up consisted of 5 minutes of arm ergometry on the Schwinn Air-Dyne. He was then instructed in use of the CES and was allowed to perform several repetitions of rotation at the various speeds to be tested.

The test consisted of five repetitions at each speed. He was noted to have a significant agonist-antagonist strength imbalance in shoulder rotation on the right at the tested speeds of 90, 120, and 240 degrees/second. The external/internal rotation peak force ratios and average force ratios are shown in Table 2.1. Further, he was noted to have a deficit in peak force and average force in external rotation on the right as compared to the left (Table 2.2).

The patient participated in rehabilitation three times weekly for 12 weeks. An exercise diskette was initially programmed for three sets of ten repetitions of external and internal rotation with a 2-second isometric contraction at the weakest point in the range of external rotation. He exercised at the same speeds as those tested.

Exercise on the Ariel CES was preceded by 10 minutes of arm ergometry on the Schwinn Air-Dyne. The patient then inserted the diskette in the diskette drive and pressed several keys to begin. He was able to proceed through the session independently. Results of average force curves were saved weekly. At the end of each set of exercise, the patient and the physical therapist could compare results with previous sessions.

At 6 weeks, the patient was tested once again on the testing diskette. Improvement was noted in external/internal rotation ratios as well as left/right external rotation ratios. Results are shown in Tables 2.3 and 2.4.

The exercise diskette was programmed at this point for three sets of ten repetitions in the variable velocity mode in external rotation. Set 1 began at 90 degrees/second, increasing linearly to 150 degrees/second through the range of external rotation. Set 2 increased from 120 degrees/second to 180 degrees/second, while set 3 increased from 180 degrees/second to 240 degrees/second. During this phase, the patient was training three

Table 2.1. Torque Ratio for Shoulder External/Internal Rotation—Initial

	90°/s	120°/s	240°/s
Peak torque	.15	.18	.20
Average torque	.18	.16	.14

Table 2.2. Torque Ratio for Right/Left Shoulder External Rotation—Initial

	90°/s	120°/s	240°/s
Peak torque	.79	.78	.72
Average torque	.73	.69	.64

Table 2.3. Torque Ratio for Shoulder External/Internal Rotation—6 Weeks

	90°/s	120°/s	240°/s
Peak torque	.40	.42	.45
Average torque	.40	.40	.39

Table 2.4. Torque Ratio for Right/Left Shoulder External Rotation—6 Weeks

	90°/s	120°/s	240°/s
Peak torque	.82	.77	.75
Average torque	.78	.73	.69

Table 2.5. Torque Ratio for Shoulder External/Internal Rotation—12 Weeks

	90°/s	120°/s	240°/s
Peak torque	.59	.62	.61
Average torque	.40	.39	.44

Table 2.6. Torque Ratio for Right/Left Shoulder External Rotation—12 Weeks

	90°/s	120°/s	240°/s
Peak torque	.96	.95	.91
Average torque	1.00	1.02	1.02

times weekly in the pool as well. He experienced only occasional pain during workouts, did not feel limited by his pain, and reported feeling stronger while swimming.

Final testing at 12 weeks showed further improvement in external/internal rotation ratios and left/right ratios as shown in Tables 2.5 and 2.6.

The patient is gradually increasing training in preparation for the upcoming competitive season. He is pleased with the results he has achieved.

REFERENCES

1. The Ariel Computerized Exercise System; the Intelligent System for Rehabilitation and Fitness . . . Product Brochure, Ariel Dynamics, Inc and Wilson Sporting Goods Co
2. Ariel GB: *Ariel Exerciser User's Manual.* Trabuco Canyon, CA, Ariel Dynamics, Inc, 1985
3. Ariel GB: Resistive training. *Clin Sports Med* 1983; 2:55–69
4. Jacobs I, Pope J: Measurement Reproducibility and Validity of a Computerized System for Muscle Strength Evaluation. Defense and Civil Institute of Environmental Medicine, Department of National Defense, Ontario, Canada, 1985
5. Watkins MP, Yorko J, Hare TW, Lowenthal DT: Ariel computerized exerciser: Reproducibility trials. Hahnemann University Hospital, Philadelphia (unpublished data)

3

Biodex System

$\mathbf{U}$ntil recently, the understanding and improvement of muscle function has been dependent upon available technology, and isotonic weight machines have been available for decades. Since the late 1960s, other systems that have been developed were capable of producing isokinetic movements, but only during concentric contractions. In the early 1980s, the limitations of these other systems inspired Richard Krukowski to reassess the concept of isokinetic exercise. This gave rise to the Biodex system (Fig. 3.1). To replace the traditional isotonic exercise routines, which involve constant weight performed at variable speeds, or isokinetic exercises limited by the functional limitations of concentric loading, low speeds, and low torques, Krukowski developed the concept of "equivalent resistance" and created a system that loads the muscle concentrically and eccentrically over the entire physiologic range of constant speeds and variable torques.

The Biodex is an isolated joint isokinetic system that enables measurement of the amount of torque produced at different velocities, thereby fulfilling the requirements of both the clinician and researcher for a muscle performance evaluation, testing, and measurement system. The Biodex system was conceived and developed to accomplish the full range of testing and training modes in a single coordinated system; it executes four kinds of testing and training modes through control of torque, position, and angular velocity during concentric or eccentric muscle loading. The major components of the Biodex system are shown in Figure 3.2: dynamometer controller; dynamometer powerhead; powerhead mount/patient restraint chair; IBM PC AT with monitor; BIOWARE software; attachments for each joint/pattern; accessory chair for testing joints other than the knee (see Fig. 3.3); instrument table; and printer.

Site requirements for the operation of the Biodex are as follows:

1. 125 VAC/60 Hz, 20 amp electrical service with 3-wire grounding; electrical service must be dedicated.
2. Ambient room temperature of 60 to 80°F (15.5 to 26.6°C) with up to 60% humidity.
3. Flooring capable of supporting 40 lb/sq-ft.
4. Access through passageway no less than 33 inches wide.
5. Low static environment (antistatic rugs or hard floor).
6. Approximately 64 sq ft (8 ft × 8 ft) of floor space for operating clearance.

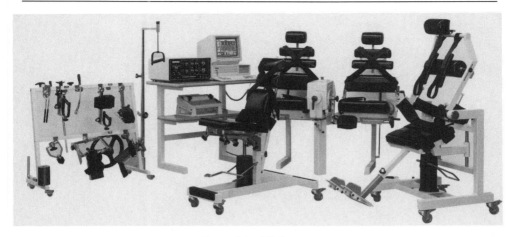

Figure 3.1. Biodex system.

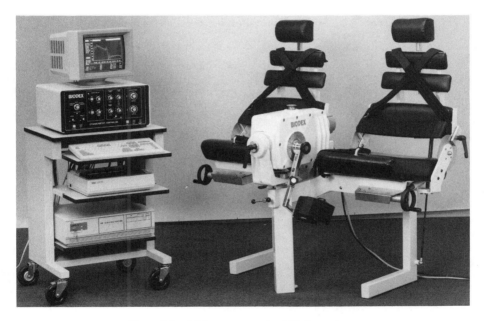

Figure 3.2. Major components of Biodex system.

The heart of the Biodex dynamometer is a torque-sensing hub assembly, attached to an output shaft of the gearbox mounted within the powerhead. The gearbox is driven by a servomotor in response to signals from a pulse-width modulated power amplifier, which in turn responds to signals from the torque-sensing hub, produced by forces applied to the output shaft by the patient.

In the isokinetic mode, precise angular velocities are attained by voltage clamping of the servomotor to a selected reference voltage. This clamped voltage signal acts

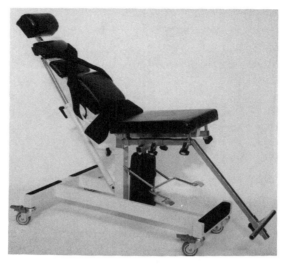

Figure 3.3.   Accessory chair for testing joints other than the knee.

as a command to the servomotor to maintain constant velocity as soon as the selected velocity is achieved. This results in an equivalent resistance, at a constant speed that cannot be exceeded, even up to 650 ft-lb of input torque.

In the eccentric mode, when a load applied to the output shaft exceeds 10% of the selected torque limit, this is sensed by the hub and causes the shaft to rotate in the direction opposite to the applied load. The instant the applied torque falls below the 10% threshold or exceeds the selected torque limit, all motions cease.

In the passive mode, the output shafts oscillate in both directions of motion at constant speed without servofeedback control. Voltage to the servomotor corresponds to the speed selected.

In the isometric mode, the output shaft is "servoed" into a static state in response to velocity voltage input from a precision tachometer.

In all modes and at any speed, any torque exerted by the patient on the powerhead shaft will be sensed by the torque hub and presented as a voltage curve on the output report.

Four Exercise Modes

The four modes of exercise that are incorporated into the Biodex are: passive, eccentric, isokinetic, and isometric resistance. The passive and eccentric modes are controlled to a constant velocity while giving accommodating resistance; therefore, they are considered to be isokinetic.

Isometric Mode

Isometric resistance is a static form of exercise that occurs when a muscle contracts without a measurable change in the length of the muscle or visible joint motion (1). By definition, no physical work occurs with an isometric contraction; however, a large amount of tension is produced by the muscle. Due to the lack of movement in isometrics, there are some inherent limitations:

1. Strength gains are somewhat specific to the point in the range of motion at which the tension was developed. One recent study by Knapik et al (2) demonstrated that a 20-degree physiologic overflow occurred from the specific joint angle. Therefore, when exercising isometrically, strength gains are greatest within 10 degrees of either direction at which the joint is positioned. This work gave rise to the concept of "multiple-angle isometric exercise" in which the joint can be exercised every 20 degrees throughout the range of motion, thereby strengthening throughout the entire range of motion (3).

2. Because there is little or no immediate feedback to the person exercising, motivation is difficult. In addition, the duration of the contraction is important, but difficult to monitor.

The ISOMETRIC mode on the Biodex system helps to resolve these difficulties in the following ways:

1. Exercise or testing joint angles can be precisely set for repeatability throughout the range of motion. An infinite number of stop positions can be selected throughout the range of motion.

2. Patient motivation is increased by both graphic and numerical data displayed in real time during the exercise session. This instant feedback can further encourage the patient.

Isokinetic Mode

Isokinetic exercise has been available since the late 1960s when it was introduced by James Perrine (3). Isokinetic exercise is a form of dynamic exercise in which force is exerted against a resistance of fixed speed. Resistance is accommodating and maintained at a constant velocity. The resistance will vary directly with the force being generated by the muscles to allow maximal muscle performance throughout the range of motion.

Isokinetic exercise and testing have become increasingly popular during the last decade. Principal reasons for this popularity are the ability of the dynamometer to match the resistance of the load arm to the torque produced by the patient, the ability to train muscles at specific velocities, and the ability to test dynamic muscle contractions related to function under physiologic conditions.

Unlike previous systems that required the patient to reach the preselected speed of the machine prior to meeting the resistance, the Biodex incorporates servotechnology. Simply stated, this allows the patient to meet resistance equal to what he/she is capable of producing while still controlling the speed. Once the preselected speed has been attained, the powerhead gives the appropriate resistance necessary to maintain that speed. If weakness, pain, length-tension, leverage, or other biomechanical changes occur, the resistance will accommodate to the forces being applied by the subject.

In addition to the traditional benefits of isokinetics, the Biodex provides additional features to the isokinetic concept:

1. The dynamometer controller sets limits of position over the range of motion precisely in small increments.

2. There is no possibility of setting an undesired increase in the range of motion. The input fixture is moved by the patient to the limits of his/her range of motion, and pushbuttons are pressed to set and control the range of motion limits. During the course of exercise, these range of motion (ROM) limits may be decreased by a desired percentage, but in no case may they be increased. Thus a precise and extremely safe control of range of motion is accomplished with the Biodex.

3. The Biodex controller has the capability of allowing control over acceleration and deceleration out of or into the range of motion stops so that there is a comfortable transition from dynamic to static tension and a smooth controlled reversal into the isokinetic phase of movement.

4. The Biodex system provides accurate testing results and allows exact duplication of exercise and testing movements related to precise monitoring and 23-position switch setting of speed control. An isokinetic speed of 30 to 450 degrees/second can be preselected.

The Biodex system has the ability to allow the selection of different velocities or loadings for each direction of motion. Thus it is possible to do an isokinetic concentric knee extension at 60 degrees/second and then a concentric knee flexion at 240 degrees/second. This combination of control of range of motion and control of velocity greatly expands the application to rehabilitative programs.

The angular position and velocity can be exactly duplicated with the Biodex system. Until recently, range of angular position or ROM could not be controlled, only blocked with physical stops. Speeds could be selected, but not critically controlled for acceleration and deceleration cushions.

The Biodex system is continually monitoring speed, angular position (ROM), and torque by means of sensitive, rapidly correcting comparative circuits in the dynamometer controller logic. However, with any isokinetic exercise it should be remembered that motivation plays an important role. If the user is motivated, he/she exerts sufficient force to meet the velocity at which the dynamometer is set and experiences an equivalent resistance to his/her input torque. If the user is undermotivated, he/she can continue to move through a full range of motion, at less than the selected speeds and experiencing no resistance.

Eccentric Mode

With the Biodex system, ECCENTRIC is both a mode of operation and a method of muscle loading. This eccentric mode can be described as "reactive eccentric." The eccentric mode of exercise is initiated with a premovement contraction. This means a muscular movement and loading in such a way that any force exerted by the patient is opposed by an equivalent opposite force generated by the dynamometer. The force necessary to start the movement is $1/10$ of the torque limit setting in each direction. Once the minimum threshold is attained, the shaft of the powerhead moves at a constant speed in the opposite direction of the force applied. If the applied force either drops below $1/10$ of the present torque limits or exceeds the torque limits that were selected, the powerhead will slow down and stop. Because the patient must continually meet the minimal threshold for movement to occur, the patient has the ability to cancel the movement at any time (for instance, if there is pain). Velocity of movement can range from 10 to 120 degrees/second. Torque limits can be set between the ranges of .5 to 150 ft-lb of pressure. Threshold values can be established for both directions of movement.

Passive Mode

By far the most diverse mode of exercise and its application for rehabilitation is the isokinetic passive mode. For patients who cannot produce voluntary contractions because of pain, weakness, or neurologic causes, isometric and isokinetic training and testing is beyond reach. Thus the passive mode is used for a wide variety of training and assessment protocols in acute patients. The key features of this mode are:

1. Range of motion is precisely controlled and limited by multiple safety stops.
2. Passive motion is accompanied by a fine control of cushioned electronic stops. Passive speed may be adjusted between 2 to 120 degrees/second.
3. In the passive mode, a rest interval or pause, varying from 0 to 4 seconds, may be selected between directions of motion.
4. A maximum torque level can be selected for each direction of motion. If during a passive movement the patient attempts to resist the movement with a torque greater than the preset torque limit, the load cell senses that torque and stops the motion of the load arm, giving immediate feedback that the patient is overexerting. The maximum torque limit setting is 150 ft-lb and the minimum is .5 ft-lb.

In the passive mode, the clinician is able to select combinations of concentric/concentric, eccentric/eccentric, eccentric/concentric or concentric/eccentric type of muscle contractions. Deciding on one versus another can be made easier when there is a further understanding of the capabilities of the passive mode.

Some of the physiologic and clinical applications of the passive mode on the Biodex include the following:

1. Passive motion may be used to warm-up and cool-down a patient. Used during rest periods, passive motion can help to prevent the muscles from "tightening up" before the next set.
2. When used as a modified eccentric mode, passive assist has physiologic advantages similar to eccentrics yet retains the advantages of the passive mode. Concentrate on agonist muscle groups and if necessary avoid any antagonist work simply by giving the patient specific commands. Working this way will provide a concentric and eccentric contraction of the same muscle group.
3. In the case of poor muscle strength, passive motion will initiate or continue motion of the patient. Because full range of motion and movement against gravity are not required, it is not necessary for a patient to have a minimal level of muscle strength to start using the Biodex.
4. If a portion of the range of motion is painful, a cooperative patient can exercise up to the start of the painful range, let up the resistance causing a passive move-

ment through the painful range, and resume active exercise when out of the painful arc.

5. Muscle relaxation deficits can be treated by using the pause control and descending from 4 to 1 second, allowing less time for the patient to react to movement.

6. Through trial repetitions, calculate the maximum concentric capability. Use the torque limit dials to set the eccentric forces so they do not exceed the concentric forces.

7. Passive motion can be used for gradual increase in range of motion with patients for whom it is restricted.

Reliability and Validity

The torque channel of the Biodex system utilizes an assembly of strain gauges to measure torsional loads on the powerhead's shaft. This load cell is an integral part of the shaft assembly, monitoring rotational forces about the physiologic axis aligned with the shaft during the setup. This placement of the load cell ensures against torque errors associated with designs that correlate force measurements taken elsewhere in the mechanical system with torque at the primary shaft. The Biodex torque signal is not subject to errors resulting from variables such as velocity-induced and thermal-induced changes in mechanical efficiency, and the signal requires no mechanical or electronic damping at any point in the system.

Strain gauges are an ideal choice in torque measurement because of their high linearity and durability. The gauges selected for use in the Biodex have a yield point corresponding to 1600 ft-lb of torque at the powerhead shaft. This means that signal error or loss resulting from overstressing a strain gauge would require exceeding the 450 ft-lb rating of the system by more than 1000 ft-lb. Because the Biodex utilizes multiple gauges arranged in a bridge, failure of any single gauge would be recognized by the circuit's logic, causing the system to shutdown and display "STRAIN GAUGE LOSS" on the powerhead's diagnostic panel.

When an attachment approaches a preset electronic stop, a substantial torque is often generated as the arm "bounces" off the stop. Because of the great sensitivity of the strain gauge circuit, these "isometric" torque signals are recorded along with the torque signals generated during the isokinetic study. The signals are referred to as "isometric contractions" because they occur when the attachment is at zero velocity. Because isokinetic testing presupposes that torque is produced at a constant velocity, these isometric contractions are technically "nonisokinetic" and therefore should not make contributions to measurements of peak torque, position, work, or power. The Clinical Data Station automatically eliminates isometric contractions during the isokinetic test procedure. The attachment is considered at "zero" velocity when moving less than 5 degrees/second. This "threshold" minimizes the occurrence of false starts and assures that acquisition does not begin until the attachment is actually in motion.

To date, there has been no published research on the clinical reliability and validity of the data provided by the Biodex system. Several investigations are currently underway to assess the accuracy of both velocity of movement and torque values produced. Repeated clinical trials using a known weight at a fixed distance from the torque sensing hub assembly resulted in a 99% accuracy percentage when using the

Bioware software program for data acquisition. The Biodex powerhead is factory calibrated to a standard that assures accuracy of the torque signal to within ±0.5%.

Biodex Acquisition Software

The Biodex software package is a collection of programs for acquisition, display, processing, and reporting of studies performed on the Biodex. The Clinical Data Station supplied with the system provides data storage up to 20 megabytes, with Enhanced Graphics, 640k memory, and 10 mHz processor. The software package allows the clinician to perform the following tasks:

Data Collection

Four possible "real time" signals are acquired and stored by the acquisition software: TORQUE, POSITION, VELOCITY, and ELAPSED TIME. Torque is defined as force applied over a rotational distance from a single "center point," namely the shaft axis. Torque is measured in units of foot-pounds (ft-lb). Position is an angular measurement of the current anatomical position of the joint relative to anatomical zero. Position is measured in degrees. Velocity is the angular velocity of the joint and is measured in degrees per second (deg/sec). Elapsed time is measurement of the total exercise time from start to end of a single set of repetitions. Elapsed time is measured in seconds.

Data or Curve Analysis

A comprehensive data analysis program is incorporated into the Biodex acquisition software. This allows the clinician to analyze the acquired data "point by point" giving torque, position, velocity, and elapsed time for each specific point.

Report Generation

A set of detailed report formats are included with the software package; these allow the clinician to obtain a printed record of the patient's progress during rehabilitation.

Rehabilitation Protocol

Included in the Biodex software is a section that allows the operator total control of the rehabilitative process while providing the patient with motivating biofeedback.

Data Collection

After patient records have been established, a menu of procedures will appear on the computer screen. A tester may select from one of the following:

System Calibration

The system calibration protocol instructs the operator to make the measurements necessary for calibration of the Biodex system. The measurements assure that the system is calibrated for accurate position and torque measurements. If at any time the calibration factors become invalid, a warning message will appear until the calibration factors are within tolerance.

Verify Calibration

The quality assurance protocol offers a fast, convenient method of assuring the reliability and integrity of position, torque, and velocity measurements made with the Biodex system. This protocol produces a real-time display of the current load arm position, torque, and corresponding velocity values being measured.

Clinical Two-Speed Bilateral Test

This protocol is designed to conduct a bilateral test on the selected joint using the specified test pattern. The study consists of four data sets: two sets collected at slow and fast speed on the uninvolved side and two sets collected on the involved side. Prior to testing, the system must be calibrated to joint angle and weight of the limb.

Clinical Three-Speed Bilateral Test

In this protocol, three speeds can be selected for testing.

Velocity Spectrum Protocol Testing

This program allows for six-speed unilateral testing of a specific joint pattern.

Exercise Protocol

The exercise rehabilitation protocol is designed to conduct exercise sessions oriented toward rehabilitation. Exercise bouts can be arranged in sets of repetitions, time, or total work. In this mode, data are not saved on the hard disk; however, a hard copy can be printed during the course of the exercise session. The main function of this program is providing motivational feedback utilizing graphics and sound to prompt the patient through the exercise bouts.

Once a test protocol has been completed, the software returns the user to the Biodex home menu. The user can then select curve analysis or can choose to have a report printed. There are four basic reports that the clinician can select: (1) Comprehensive report (Fig. 3.4)—a detailed analysis of each evaluation session with medicolegal acceptance (as with all Biodex output reports); (2) Bilateral summary (Fig. 3.5)—a concise comparison of the functional abilities of the uninjured limb and the injured limb; (3) Velocity spectrum summary (Fig. 3.6)—a unilateral analysis of the limb's ability to perform work at varying speeds; and (4) Referral summary (Fig. 3.7)—a bilateral summary simplified for the referring physician.

In addition to the above reports, the user may select a cumulative progress report (Figs. 3.8 and 3.9). In the exercise mode, a report can be printed simultaneous with exercise and added to the patient's chart, thereby allowing the clinician to monitor progress on a daily basis.

The curve analysis program allows the clinician interactive analysis of torque, position, and velocity data acquired from the Biodex test protocol. Individual repetitions can be displayed on the screen. Depending on the current curve mode, torque, position, or velocity data will be displayed. This program allows for information to appear as an overlay on the screen for comparative purposes. Cursors can be superimposed over the curve data and move to any point along the curve. Wherever the cursors lie, the corresponding time, torque, position, and velocity information for that point

```
                                    Aug 03, 1987 at 11:00:54
                    BIODEX COMPREHENSIVE REPORT
                    ***************************
```

```
Name      : AB                   Joint         : KNEE
ID        : 0991                 Pattern       : Extension/Flexion
Date      : Jun 16, 1987         Involved Side : L
Age       : 23                   Settings      : 34.5\ 14.5\ 5
Sex       : M                    Injury/Surgery: 2\ 14\ 86
Height    : 75                   Calibration   : Jul 31, 1987 16:41:55
Weight    : 225                  Mode          : Isokinetic
Clinician : TB                   Contraction   : Concentric/Concentric
Referral  : Walsh
```

```
UNINJURED Side :  5.00 Repetitions Acquired at   60.0/  60.0 deg/sec
```

Measurement	Extension	Flexion	Ratio
Peak Torque:	248.0 ft-lbs	164.0 ft-lbs	66.1 %
Peak Torque "Rep":	2.00	1.00	
Time to Peak Torque:	0.42 secs	0.35 secs	
Angle of Peak Torque:	80.0 degs	35.0 degs	
Torque @ 30.0 deg:	57.0 ft-lbs	148.0 ft-lbs	
Torque @ 0.20 sec:	208.0 ft-lbs	143.0 ft-lbs	
Torque / Body Weight:	110.2 %	72.9 %	
Work / Body Weight:	94.6 %	74.3 %	
Max Rep Work:	212.8 ft-lbs	167.2 ft-lbs	78.6 %
Max Work "Rep":	2.00	1.00	
Total Work:	996.9 ft-lbs	769.1 ft-lbs	77.1 %
Work First Third:	206.3 ft-lbs	167.2 ft-lbs	81.1 %
Work Last Third:	177.5 ft-lbs	135.2 ft-lbs	81.1 %
Work Fatigue:	13.9 %	19.1 %	
Average Power:	134.5 watts	97.2 watts	

```
        Maximum ROM:     94.0 deg, from  14.0 to 109.0 degs
        Maximum GET:     15.0 ft-lbs
```

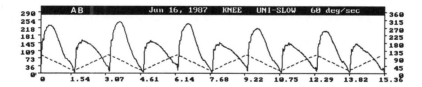

Figure 3.4. Comprehensive report.

in the study will be displayed on the screen below the graphic window. A graphic snapshot of the curve analysis displayed on the screen can be generated at any time.

Clinical Application

Clinical application of the Biodex begins with a thorough understanding of the dynamometer controller (Fig. 3.10). Once the system has been turned on, the user then selects the desired mode of operation. During the initial setup, the machine can-

```
                                        Aug 03, 1987 at 11:05:20
                        BIODEX BILATERAL SUMMARY
                        *************************

       Name      : A B            Joint         : KNEE
       ID        : 0991           Pattern       : Extension/Flexion
       Date      : Jun 16, 1987   Involved Side : L
       Age       : 23             Settings      : 34.5\ 14.5\ 5
       Sex       : M              Injury/Surgery: 2\ 14\ 86
       Height    : 75             Calibration   : Jul 31, 1987 16:41:55
       Weight    : 225            Mode          : Isokinetic
       Clinician : TB             Contraction   : Concentric/Concentric
       Referral  : Walsh
```

SLOW Speed : 5.00 Repetitions Acquired at   60.0/ 60.0 deg/sec

Extension	Uninjured	Injured	Deficit
Peak Torque:	248.0 ft-lbs	201.0 ft-lbs	19.0 %
Time to Peak Torque:	0.42 secs	0.40 secs	-4.76 %
Max Rep Work:	212.8 ft-lbs	172.2 ft-lbs	19.1 %
Total Work:	996.9 ft-lbs	817.1 ft-lbs	18.0 %

Flexion	Uninjured	Injured	Deficit
Peak Torque:	164.0 ft-lbs	137.0 ft-lbs	16.5 %
Time to Peak Torque:	0.35 secs	0.34 secs	-2.86 %
Max Rep Work:	167.2 ft-lbs	140.8 ft-lbs	15.8 %
Total Work:	769.1 ft-lbs	649.0 ft-lbs	15.6 %
Maximum ROM:	94.0 deg	94.0 deg	%
Anatomical ROM:	14.0 to 109.0	12.0 to 106.0 degs	

FAST Speed : 10.0 Repetitions Acquired at 180.0/ 180.0 deg/sec

Extension	Uninjured	Injured	Deficit
Peak Torque:	157.0 ft-lbs	147.0 ft-lbs	6.37 %
Time to Peak Torque:	0.19 secs	0.11 secs	-42.1 %
Max Rep Work:	47.1 ft-lbs	40.3 ft-lbs	14.5 %
Total Work:	421.8 ft-lbs	356.8 ft-lbs	15.4 %

Flexion	Uninjured	Injured	Deficit
Peak Torque:	137.0 ft-lbs	119.0 ft-lbs	13.1 %
Time to Peak Torque:	0.09 secs	0.12 secs	33.3 %
Max Rep Work:	38.8 ft-lbs	31.9 ft-lbs	17.8 %
Total Work:	345.0 ft-lbs	296.6 ft-lbs	14.0 %
Maximum ROM:	95.0 deg	95.0 deg	%
Anatomical ROM:	14.0 to 109.0	10.0 to 106.0 degs	

Figure 3.5. Bilateral summary.

not be engaged without first setting the range of motion (ROM) safety limits in the SetUp mode. After the ROM limits have been set, the clinician can then switch to the desired mode. Designed into the electronics of the mode setting switch are prompting lights which assist the clinician in proper setup prior to engaging the desired mode of operation. When setting the mode switch to the following modes of operation, specific lights will illuminate, indicating to the operator the functions that must be selected for that mode to operate as desired by the clinician:

Aug 06, 1987 at 12:12:33

BIODEX VELOCITY SPECTRUM EVALUATION
****

Name : T.B.	Joint	: KNEE
ID : 0991	Pattern	: Extension/Flexion
Date : Jun 16, 1987	Involved Side	: L
Age : 23	Settings	: 34.5
Sex : M	Injury/Surgery:	none
Height : 75	Calibration	: Jul 31, 1987 16:41:55
Weight : 225	Mode	: Isokinetic
Clinician: T.S.	Contraction	: Concentric/Concentric
Referral : Walsh		

Extension

Speed	# Reps	Peak Torque	Max Rep Work	Total Work	Ave Power
60.0/ 60.0 d/s	5.00	191.0 ft-lbs	172.2 ft-lbs	831.7 ft-lbs	111.6 wts
90.0/ 90.0 d/s	5.00	178.0 ft-lbs	115.1 ft-lbs	550.9 ft-lbs	104.7 wts
120.0/ 120.0 d/s	5.00	166.0 ft-lbs	79.9 ft-lbs	376.9 ft-lbs	92.4 wts
150.0/ 150.0 d/s	5.00	151.0 ft-lbs	55.4 ft-lbs	259.9 ft-lbs	79.2 wts
180.0/ 180.0 d/s	5.00	136.0 ft-lbs	42.9 ft-lbs	197.2 ft-lbs	70.2 wts
210.0/ 210.0 d/s	5.00	137.0 ft-lbs	33.4 ft-lbs	157.6 ft-lbs	65.7 wts

Flexion

Speed	# Reps	Peak Torque	Max Rep Work	Total Work	Ave Power
60.0/ 60.0 d/s	5.00	136.0 ft-lbs	143.2 ft-lbs	676.5 ft-lbs	86.8 wts
90.0/ 90.0 d/s	5.00	138.0 ft-lbs	94.6 ft-lbs	445.4 ft-lbs	81.6 wts
120.0/ 120.0 d/s	5.00	139.0 ft-lbs	67.0 ft-lbs	306.0 ft-lbs	72.9 wts
150.0/ 150.0 d/s	5.00	119.0 ft-lbs	45.9 ft-lbs	223.2 ft-lbs	66.4 wts
180.0/ 180.0 d/s	5.00	124.0 ft-lbs	36.6 ft-lbs	178.2 ft-lbs	63.0 wts
210.0/ 210.0 d/s	5.00	137.0 ft-lbs	32.4 ft-lbs	151.6 ft-lbs	61.6 wts

Figure 3.6. Velocity spectrum summary.

Mode of Operation

Passive

Passive speed light and torque limit light will illuminate, indicating that the proper speed and the desired torque should be selected.

Eccentric

Eccentric speed light and torque limit light will illuminate, indicating that the proper speed for both directions of motion, and the desired torque limits for each direction of motion independently, should be selected.

Isokinetic

Isokinetic speed light will illuminate indicating that the desired speed for each direction of movement should be selected.

Isometric

No light will illuminate because isometric means zero speed of operation. No speed or torque selections need to be made. The ROM limits must be pressed to change the joint angle as desired.

```
                                          Aug 03, 1987 at 11:07:41
                        BIODEX REFERRAL SUMMARY
                        ***********************

      Name      : A B              Joint         : KNEE
      ID        : 0991             Pattern       : Extension/Flexion
      Date      : Jun 16, 1987     Involved Side : L
      Age       : 23               Settings      : 34.5\ 14.5\ 5
      Sex       : M                Injury/Surgery: 2\ 14\ 86
      Height    : 75               Calibration   : Jul 31, 1987 16:41:55
      Weight    : 225              Mode          : Isokinetic
      Clinician: TB                Contraction   : Concentric/Concentric
      Referral : Walsh
```

	SLOW Speed : 5.00 Reps at 60.0/ 60.0 deg/sec			FAST Speed : 10.0 Reps at 180.0/ 180.0 deg/sec		
Extension	Uninjured	Injured	Deficit	Uninjured	Injured	Deficit
Peak Torque:	248.0 ft-lbs	201.0 ft-lbs	19.0 %	157.0 ft-lbs	147.0 ft-lbs	6.37 %
Time to Peak Torque:	0.42 secs	0.40 secs	-4.76 %	0.19 secs	0.11 secs	-42.1 %
Max Rep Work:	212.8 ft-lbs	172.2 ft-lbs	19.1 %	47.1 ft-lbs	40.3 ft-lbs	14.5 %
Flexion	Uninjured	Injured	Deficit	Uninjured	Injured	Deficit
Peak Torque:	164.0 ft-lbs	137.0 ft-lbs	16.5 %	137.0 ft-lbs	119.0 ft-lbs	13.1 %
Time to Peak Torque:	0.35 secs	0.34 secs	-2.86 %	0.09 secs	0.12 secs	33.3 %
Max Rep Work:	167.2 ft-lbs	140.8 ft-lbs	15.8 %	38.8 ft-lbs	31.9 ft-lbs	17.8 %
Maximum ROM:	94.0 deg	94.0 deg	%	95.0 deg	95.0 deg	%
Anatomical ROM:	14.0 to 109.0	12.0 to 106.0		14.0 to 109.0	10.0 to 106.0 degs	
Maximum GET:	15.0 ft-lbs	17.0 ft-lbs				

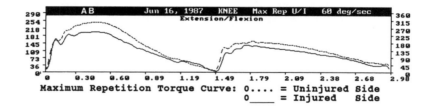

Maximum Repetition Torque Curve: 0.... = Uninjured Side
                                  0____ = Injured   Side

Definition of Parameters

Peak Torque   — Highest torque developed in a set
Time to Peak Torque — Indicator of the functional ability
                       to produce torque quickly
Max Rep Work   — Measurement of the maximum work produced
                       in a single repetition
Max ROM   — Maximum range of motion for the indicated
                       joint test pattern

*** BIODEX Corporate Office ***

Figure 3.7. Referral summary.

The LOAD ARM INDICATOR functions to indicate the direction in which force is being applied to the Biodex input arm. The Biodex incorporates a torque sensing circuit in its system. This circuit allows clinical measurement of torques as low as 1 ft-lb with an error of less than 2%. When an individual is using the system and applies force to the dynamometer by means of the proper input accessory, one of the red load arm indicator lights will illuminate, displaying the direction of movement (the force) is

Aug 03, 1987 at 11:08:49

BIODEX PROGRESS REPORT
****

CURRENT PATIENT IMFORMATION

Name	: A B	Joint	: KNEE
ID	: 0991	Pattern	: Extension/Flexion
Date	: Jun 16, 1987	Involved Side	: L
Age	: 23	Settings	: 34.5\ 14.5\ 5
Sex	: M	Injury/Surgery	: 2\ 14\ 86
Height	: 75	Calibration	: Jul 31, 1987 16:41:55
Weight	: 225		
Mode	: Isokinetic	Contraction	: Concentric/Concentric
Referral	: Walsh	Clinician	: TB

COMPARATIVE PATIENT IMFORMATION

Name	: DE	Joint	: KNEE
ID	:	Pattern	: Extension/Flexion
Date	: May 26, 1987	Involved Side	: L
Age	: 38	Settings	: 32.5;11.52.5;3
Sex	: F	Injury/Surgery	: 2-23-84
Height	: 66	Calibration	: Jul 31, 1987 16:41:55
Weight	: 126		
Mode	: Isokinetic	Contraction	: Concentric/Concentric
Referral	: TEMPLE	Clinician	: CLEMMER

Progress Statistics Summary

	Peak Torque Extension	Peak Torque Flexion	Time to Peak Torque Extension	Time to Peak Torque Flexion	Max Rep Work Extension	Max Rep Work Flexion	Max Range of Motion
UNI-SLOW Set :	-195%	-228%	22%	13%	-140%	-185%	1%
UNI-FAST Set :	-196%	-291%	41%	68%	-101%	-117%	0%
INJ-SLOW Set :	-224%	-204%	26%	42%	-166%	-198%	-6%
INJ-FAST Set :	-133%	-240%	54%	0%	-54%	-92%	-7%

COMMENTS:

Figure 3.8. Progress report with statistics summary.

being applied. When the center green light is illuminated, it means that no force is being applied in either direction.

The CUSHION switch sets the "softness" of the selected range of motion stops. The dynamometer controller limits the subject's range of motion by signaling the powerhead to prevent further shaft rotation when a preset range limit has been raised. To avoid subject discomfort or trauma to a joint, the shaft is stopped by a smooth deceleration as the range limit is approached. The cushion adjustment dial provides a means of varying the point at which deceleration starts. When a "hard" cushion is selected, deceleration begins relatively close to the stopping point. When a "soft" cushion setting is used, deceleration begins earlier. The cushion is actually slowing the speed at which you are moving, in much the same way as the braking mechanism on a car slows the car down. It is not absorbing an inpact, but rather bringing the input arm and limb to a comfortable rate of stopping.

Aug 03, 1987 at 11:08:52

BIODEX PROGRESS REPORT
****

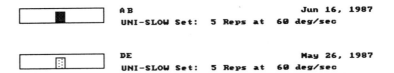

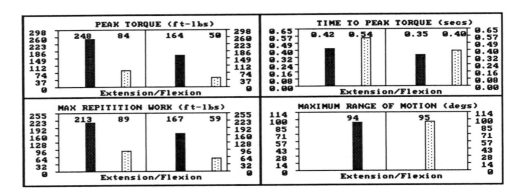

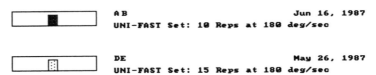

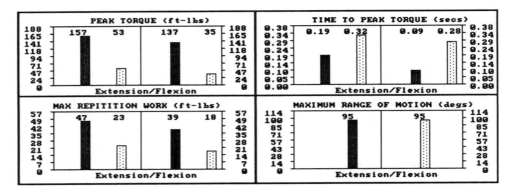

Figure 3.9. Progress report with bar graph comparisons.

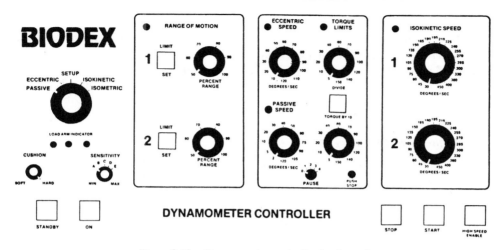

Figure 3.10. Dynamometer controller front panel.

The SENSITIVITY switch sets the torque threshold necessary to initiate movement of each Biodex input accessory. Because each accessory piece weighs a different amount, it is necessary to select the level of sensitivity that will lower the torque threshold in order to initiate a pattern of movement. The proper sensitivity setting is engraved on each Biodex fixture.

Range of Motion Limits

This functions to set the maximum allowable ROM. Multiple safety circuits monitor each other constantly. If for any reason one or both circuits malfunction, the input arm would come to a complete stop. The dynamometer cannot be engaged in a selected mode without first setting the range of motion limits in each direction. The range of motion percent range dials allow the clinician to set a specific ROM within the maximum limit set. Adjustments can be made from 50% to 100% of the maximum safety limits set for directions 1 and 2.

Eccentric Mode

In this mode, the powerhead responds to torque input by rotating the shaft in an opposing direction at a constant velocity (eccentric speed dial controls the angular velocity from a minimum of 10 degrees/second to a maximum of 120 degrees/second). In this mode, the torque limit adjustment dials are used to specify a range of desired human force output. To induce shaft motion, the subject is required to exceed a minimum torque threshold corresponding to 10% of the torque limit dial settings. If the exercise subject exceeds the torque limit value selected for either direction of motion, the shaft stops rotating until the subject's force output is reduced to within the desired range. The subject is therefore required (1) to exceed one specific torque value to achieve motion and (2) to keep torque output below another specified level to continue movement.

Passive Mode

In this mode, the powerhead provides continuous motion at constant velocity, with direction changes occurring only when range-of-motion limits are reached. Passive speed can be set at a minimum of 2 degrees/second to a maximum speed of 120 degrees/second. When the start button is pressed to initiate exercise in this mode, shaft velocity increases gradually over a period of 10 seconds, safely and comfortably bringing the subject up to exercise speed.

High-Speed Enable

This button flashes when a starting speed of 60 degrees/second or higher is selected in the passive or eccentric mode. To begin exercise when this condition exists, the operator must depress the "Start" and "High Speed Enable" buttons simultaneously. This feature is designed to caution against initiating shaft motion at a speed that may be too high for a particular individual or pattern of exercise.

The PAUSE sets the time interval before the input accessory will change directions when the passive mode is selected. Zero pause means that there is no time interval before changing directions and that the unit will operate in a continuous passive motion mode.

The following joint movement patterns are supported by the Biodex system:

1. Shoulder abduction/adduction
2. Shoulder flexion/extension
3. Shoulder internal/external rotation
4. Shoulder abduction-flexion/adduction-extension
5. Elbow flexion/extension
6. Forearm supination/pronation
7. Wrist flexion/extension
8. Wrist radial/ulnar deviation
9. Knee extension/flexion
10. Knee tibial internal/external rotation
11. Ankle dorsiflexion/plantarflexion
12. Ankle eversion/inversion
13. Back extension/flexion (with accessory system)
14. Customized tests for any hand motion

Patient setup into a desired joint test or exercise position is conveniently made through a minimal number of attachments (Fig. 3.1). In addition to the standard attachments, optional accessories for back testing, work hardening, sliding cuff for patellofemoral, and an antishear pad for ACL patients are available.

Application of the Biodex system into patient care is diverse through the different modes of operation. The device can be used in the isometric or passive modes with the acute care patient or postoperative patient, and the device can be used throughout the rehabilitation program with functional training. An example of the variability of the Biodex system is presented in the following case history in which the Biodex was used from the beginning and throughout the entire rehabilitation program.

Case Study

The patient was a 24-year-old female intercollegiate soccer player who ruptured her anterior cruciate ligament while being tackled from behind. An intra-articular repair was performed utilizing a patellar tendon allograft. Following surgery, the lower extremity was placed into a long leg immobilizer. The patient was given crutches and instructed to remain NWB (non-weight-bearing). Postoperative rehabilitation progress is summarized below:

Week 3: Physical Therapy Ordered. Patient was initiated onto a partial weight-bearing gait pattern. Range of motion was: active, 0 to 80; passive, 0 to 90. Biodex program was: passive mode through the full available range of motion with a 4-second pause at the end range of motion. Hamstring musculature was initiated onto submaximal eccentric program building to maximal voluntary eccentric loading.

Week 4: Range of Motion: Active, 0 to 120; Passive, 0 to 125. Patient was allowed to begin full weight-bearing (FWB) without assistive device as she has demonstrated a gait pattern without deviation. Stability remains unchanged as measured by KT-1000. No pivot shift.

Week 6. Isometric quadricep work was initiated at 40 degrees of knee flexion. Biodex rehabilitation protocol setup for 10 sets of 10 repetitions times a 10-second hold. Patient continues on eccentric hamstring program: 5 sets of 2500 ft-lb total work.

Week 8: Range of Motion Now Within Normal Limits. Stability remains unchanged. Patient continues on 40 degree isometric quadricep work and eccentric hamstring program.

Week 10: Submaximal Isokinetic Quadricep Work Initiated Within Range of 90 to 40 Degrees. Over the next 6-week period, both the intensity and ROM were progressively increased to full ROM with maximal effort. A velocity spectrum protocol from 60 to 450 degrees/second was utilized with the rehabilitation program set to elapsed time of 30 seconds on followed by a 45-second rest period. The patient continued on the eccentric hamstring program.

Week 17. Isokinetic testing demonstrated the following comparative statistics: At 60 degrees/second: 15% quadricep deficit on the left; left hamstrings graded 7% stronger. At 240 degrees/second: 3% quadricep deficit on the left; left hamstrings graded 8% stronger. No change in the patient's stability.

Week 18. The patient was discharged to an independent home program. A progressive running program was initiated.

Week 24. Isokinetic testing demonstrated no deficit. Patient has returned to running without complication. Stability remains unchanged as measured by KT-1000.

Week 36. No change in isokinetic or stability testing.

Restoring Work Skills

Another rehabilitative area in which the Biodex system can be utilized is in the emerging pursuit of work hardening. The Biodex Work Simulation set provides a means of therapy for restoration of workplace skills and dexterity impaired by disease or injury of the upper extremities. Conventional exercise equipment does not adequately reproduce complex workplace motions encountered in everyday life. Shop equipment is too specialized, costly, and bulky for the physical therapy office and falls short of preparing the patient for performing actual tasks that would be encountered while on the job.

The work simulation set provides numerous applications related to the simulation of job tasks and upper extremity movements. Use of the tools works range of motion, upper extremity strength, and fatigue tolerance. The Biodex system allows the therapist to monitor thoroughly the patient's progress on the job task for rapid return to function. The work simulation set aids in recreating the patient's occupational activities and measures his/her level of performance.

All of the work simulation motions can be accomplished in isokinetic, passive, eccentric, or isometric modes at speeds up to 450 degrees/second and torques up to 450 ft-lb in the isokinetic mode. All of the speed, torque, and safety features are identical with those of the Biodex multijoint system. All of the motions can be tested and documented for medicolegal or diagnostic purposes using the software package.

Realistic simulation of certain motions can be achieved by taking advantage of the different modes of operation on the Biodex. For example, in the eccentric mode, with the powerhead tilted to 30 degrees and using an eccentric speed of 40 degrees/ second, the steering wheel attachment feels like it is attached to the steering post of a tractor trailer being driven down an interstate highway. Another example of work simulation would be using the breaker bar in the isokinetic mode with the powerhead tilted 45 degrees. With direction 1 speed set at 300 degrees/second and direction 2 speed set at 30 degrees/second, the patient experiences the sensation of tightening a large threaded bolt.

Through continual refinement, the Biodex Corporation constantly strives to increase the quality and value of its multijoint system. By using the latest technology, Biodex has produced new attachments that directly address the growing interest of rehabilitation professionals in areas such as hip testing, lift simulation, back testing, and systems to provide objective orthopedic evaluation. In the future, Biodex Corporation is committed to building attachments compatible with the existing dynamometer, thus ensuring that the Biodex user can take advantage of new attachments to cover most clinical needs.

REFERENCES

1. Lehmkuhl LD, Smith LK: *Brunstrom's Clinical Kinesiology,* ed 4. Philadelphia, FA Davis, 1983
2. Knapik JJ, Mawdley RH, Ramos MV et al: Angular specificity and test mode specificity of isometric and isokinetic strength training. *J Orthop Sports Phys Ther* 1983; 5:58–65
3. Davies G: *A Compendium of Isokinetics in Clinical Usage,* ed 2., LaCrosse, WI, S & S Publishers, 1985

4

Cybex 340 Isokinetic Rehabilitation and Testing System

The Cybex 340 is the newly released isokinetic system that is a multiple step up from the older model, the Cybex II+. The system includes improved computer enhancement, electronics, mechanical features, and stabilization. The Cybex 340 software now gives the clinician clinical information in color graphic form with speed, versatility, and multiple capabilities.

The new, contemporary design features a double-seated unit for the testing and/or exercise of knees/ankles, dynamometer, variable position color monitor, and keyboard and clinical work station with printer and accessories cabinet—all attached to a single base (Fig. 4.1). The Upper-Body Exercise and Testing Table (UBXT) is the only separate piece for testing or exercising the upper and lower extremities, allowing for 18 different joint patterns.

The major electronic components are housed in the Clinical Work Station (CWS). Contained within the CWS is the advanced power sequencer, isolation transformer, speed controller, an IBM AT compatible computer with 30-megabyte hard drive, 1.2-megabyte floppy drive with 60-megabyte streamer tape backup, system status and diagnostic module, manual system override module, and an optional uninterruptable power source.

The advanced power sequencer selectively controls the distribution of power to the system in a logical manner when powering the unit up or down. While the unit is on, it provides protection against ratio frequency and electromagnetic interference and protection against power surges and transient suppression. The unique feature of powering the unit down consists of the automatic tape backup of daily data and clinical information changes.

The speed controller accurately controls the dynamometer speed. The speeds may be selected at the speed controller itself or from the keyboard when in computer mode. The speed is controlled through digital signals ensuring precise accurate settings from 0 to 300 degrees/second. The speed increments are as before: 0, 30, 45, 60, 75, 90, 105, 120, 135, 150, 180, 210, 240, 270, and 300 degrees/second. In addition, 12 degrees/second is also available during weighing of the limb, which is the optimal limb weighing speed for maximum accuracy in determining the gravity effect torque.

There is also the feature of time-based acceleration ramping. When a specific

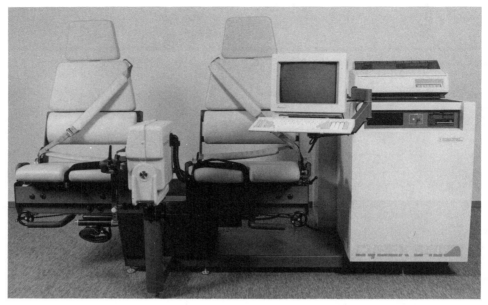

Figure 4.1. Cybex 340 Isokinetic Rehabilitation and Testing System. Photograph courtesy of Cybex.

acceleration ramp is selected and activated and force is applied to the dynamometer, the patient is allowed to accelerate the limb from a preset low speed (including zero, an isometric premovement contraction) to a preselected final exercise speed in a specific amount of time. The electronic components have a structure similar to that of previous units, i.e., speeds and ramping but with the improved technology for safety and convenience.

What makes this unit different is the fully integrated computer system. The 340 has a complete system control/data processing center. The computer contains a high performance/high reliability 30-megabyte hard drive, which provides enough data storage and data management capacity for at least 1,000 pages of patient information including tests and records. One of the most unique features of the system is the streamer tape backup system. On most systems, a floppy disk backup routine must be initiated manually on a regular basis to eliminate the possibility of losing data related to power failures or surges. The 340 system automatically backs up the day's information whenever it is placed into a power-down mode. This ensures that a duplicate copy of the database is available. This will also allow for an unlimited patient data base by archiving discharged patients.

As an added feature, there is a 1.2-megabyte floppy disk drive. This will be convenient if multiple IBM-compatible units are in the office or if a clinician wishes to transfer a patient's records to a portable medium or another 1.2-megabyte floppy disk. Another option is the use of commercially available IBM-compatible software for office management work, i.e., word processing or billing.

Along with new technology come the increased possibilities of system and/or component failures. The system contains internal diagnostics which are displayed by

LCD (liquid crystal display) on the face of the clinical work station. This is the system status and diagnostics module. When there is an operation problem, this module will assist in product service.

Stationed on a variable position arm is the Mitsubishi color graphics monitor and keyboard. The arm allows easy visual and manual access to the monitor and keyboard by the patient exercising or by the clinician. The clarity and positioning should lead to excellent patient/therapist feedback. The printer, which operates with moderate speed but excellent clarity and color graphics, sits atop the CWS for easy access and paper loading.

An option that is highly recommended is the uninterruptable power source (UPS). The UPS will automatically activate in the event of a power outage, shortage or line surge. The UPS will also sustain normal operation for 15 minutes. This is enough time to complete a test and store the data or perform a tape backup.

A comforting aspect to the introduction of all this new technology is the manual system override module. As many therapists are quickly learning, in certain situations, it is appropriate to control the system in manual mode "like the good old days." By changing to manual control mode, the dynamometer speeds can be changed manually, in the event the computer cannot be used, or if the clinician chooses to exercise without computer enhancement.

This system remains isokinetic and entirely passive. The velocity is 0 to 300 degrees/second with torque measurements up to 360 ft-lb. There continues to be mechanical range limiting along with manual adjustments of the dynamometer head but with greater ease.

Because there have been no major changes in the mechanical aspects of the dynamometer, the same accuracy and reliability can be expected as in the past (1–11).

New to the extremity dynamometer is the optical encoder which provides accuracy of range of motion data within 1 degree. The dynamometer is also an integral part of the sturdy seat frame, a factor that improves the stability of the system. For experienced Cybex users, a major change is the lack of noise. There is now a soundproof enclosure for quieter operation.

Cybex has also made some significant improvements in its mechanical engineering and design. The seats are firm but comfortable and have excellent lumbar support. The seat backs are easily adjusted from fully upright to fully reclined to allow for various hip angles during knee exercise or to allow for alternate setups for ankle or prone positioning.

Another unique feature is the unilateral dynamometer axis alignment. Contrary to past practice, axis alignment is performed by moving the patient on the seat to the dynamometer. The tables are designed so that when positioning the patient with the anatomical axis relative to the dynamometer, both seats adjust simultaneously for efficiency in bilateral testing. All positioning is scaled to allow for reproduction of testing positions.

The stabilization, which has proven to be critical in test-retest reliability, has also been improved. There is a pelvic and shoulder harness system typical of motor vehicle style, which adds to the comfort and ease of application. The thigh strap has also been placed more distally to minimize restriction of quadriceps contractions. Another interesting attachment is the contralateral limb stabilization bar. When used, it will restrict the nontested or exercised limb from swinging forward; this should standardize testing even more. The handgrips have also been repositioned anteriorly and are composed of a comfortable grip material.

The 340 takes up a space of 104 inches by 71 inches (plus 60 inches for the UBXT). This is comparable to the older system and provides storage space for the accessories, therefore eliminating the need for a separate cart or wall space.

Significant detailed changes on patient positioning and stabilization, ease of operation and adjustability along with consistency as a measurement tool already make the 340 appealing. The software package adds even more; it provides visual feedback, data storage capabilities, and efficiency of operation.

The applications software consists of seven system modules. Each has a unique feature and may be used according to clinician/clinic needs. The Patient File and History contains pertinent clinical and biographical information which, when stored, will be on record for future office or clinical management requirements. Data shown in Figure 4.2 can be stored on a single screen.

In Test Mode, there is an option for 18 patterns with damping automatically set based on the size of the limb segment. This is consistent with past Cybex systems, allowing for valid normative data. The Patient Setup Record provides a quick reference for the sequence of a setup (a nice feature for new users) as well as a record of the patient positioning and protocol for easy reliable retesting.

Protocol selection can be made either in a cookbook fashion with standard protocols listed for each test code or, for the more experienced clinician, there are options for creating and updating custom and patient-specific protocols. The standard exercise protocols include high velocity, low velocity, and total velocity spectra. The system allows for one stored protocol under each category of custom and patient test or exercise per pattern test code. A sample protocol selection screen is shown in Figure 4.3.

The exercise mode utilizes visual biofeedback with a bright color, motivating, real-time data display. Both torque and work per repetition are displayed to either motivate increases or allow specificity.

NAME: DATE ADMITTED:
ADDRESS: SOCIAL SECURITY #:
TELEPHONE #: HOME   MEDICARE/AID #:
       WORK   INSURANCE ID #:
REFERRER: WORK COMP CLAIM #:
ADDRESS: CASE FILE #:
TELEPHONE #:   INJURY DATE: SEX:
           SURGERY DATE: HEIGHT:
INSURANCE CO: DATE OF BIRTH: WEIGHT:
ADDRESS: DOMINANT SIDE: % BODY FAT:
           ACTIVITY LEVEL:
CONTACT: INS. CO. #2:
TELEPHONE #:   ADDRESS:

TREATING   CONTACT:
CLINICIAN: TELEPHONE #:

Figure 4.2. Patient file and history stored on single screen.

		KNEE EXTENSION/FLEXION					
		Set 1	Set 2	Set 3	Set 4	Set 5	Set 6
1. STANDARD	Speed:	060	180	240	*	*	*
	Repetitions:	003	003	020	*	*	*
	Rest:	020	020	020	*	*	*
2. CUSTOM	Speed:	060	120	180	240	270	300
	Repetitions:	003	003	003	003	003	003
	Rest:	020	020	015	010	020	010
3. PATIENT	Speed:	060	090	180	*	*	*
	Repetitions:	003	003	015	*	*	*
	Rest:	020	020	020	*	*	*

Figure 4.3. Sample protocol selection screen.

The storage and printing capabilities have also been enhanced. With the 340, the clinician now has the option of displaying or printing any of a number of numeric and/or graphic reports from present or past-tested patients. This includes a patient history; initial, status or progress report; a bilateral comparison report (initially numeric report only); and a discharge report (numeric-type report only).

Data reports include torque vs position, peak torque vs speed, average power vs speed, endurance/fatigue, force reproducibility, and work recovery.

The introduction of the software package is timely; many clinicians are now more comfortable with measurements other than torque. More and more normative data are also being published to make clinical decisions easier (4, 12–22).

Calibration is still performed and verified with known weights. The procedure has been simplified by a double weight drop. The other cumbersome task that has been eliminated is the adjusting of the potentiometers. The ability to calibrate and verify calibration should remain an important factor for clinicians, especially when routine calibration should be documented for future legal testimony.

Because the 340 has not been put to the real clinical test (our use has been on demonstration unit), we can only speculate on how the unit would benefit an average caseload. In general, evaluations should be more efficient, exercise sessions should be more motivating to the patients, and reporting for both clinical and research purposes should be easier.

Back Testing, Rehabilitation, and Screening Systems

The discussion of the Cybex systems would not be complete without the overview of the two back testing and rehabilitation units: Trunk Extension/Flexion and Torso Rotation along with the LIFTASK System. Introduced in 1984 and with the start of clinical usage of production models in 1985, the back systems have become an accepted mode of evaluation and treatment of the back.

The Trunk Extension/Flexion Testing and Rehabilitation Unit (TEF) was designed to test and rehabilitate the muscles involved in daily lifting, carrying and reaching, as well as posture and movement. The patient is placed in a standing position with comfortable but firm and secure stabilization. Motor-controlled horizontal and vertical planes of adjustment are used to align a single compromise axis, nominally L5-S1, with the axis of the unit. The unit has been designed to accommodate patients ranging in height from 60 to 78 inches. Individual scales indicate relative patient positions for reproducibility in future tests and exercise sessions (Fig. 4.4).

Scapular and chest pads provide upper body stabilization and are the pads against which the patient flexes and extends. The lower body is stabilized in a 15-degree knee/hip flexed position by tibial, popliteal, and thigh pads, and a pelvic belt. This positioning and stabilization has proven to be functional and safe and can be reproduced accurately.

The input assembly is made of a custom alloy for low inertia and strength enabling both normal and deconditioned patients to be tested and exercised. The range of motion is limited mechanically by compression stops. These are individually adjusted to allow anywhere from -15 degrees of extension to 95 degrees of flexion. Five degrees of motion is used by the stops to decelerate the trunk in each direction. Similar to extremity testing and exercise, the range-limiting devices can be used to limit painful ranges or to allow performance of short arc or full arc motions. To aid patients who have difficulty moving from flexion into extension, a low inertia counterbalance mech-

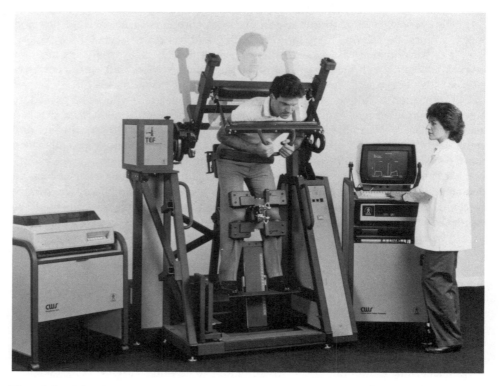

Figure 4.4. Cybex Trunk Extension/Flexion Testing and Rehabilitation Unit (TEF). Photograph courtesy of Cybex.

anism may be engaged. This mechanism has been designed to negate the effects of gravity, therefore assisting in extension. This has proven helpful for the patient with subacute or severe debilitating chronic back pain; such patients may have extremely weak or poorly functioning back extensors.

The TEF mechanical setup procedure is simple and visual computer prompts can be used. Eleven steps are required:

1. Have the patient stand face forward on the foot tray.
2. Align the vertical axis of rotation.
3. Fasten the pelvic belt.
4. Center the popliteal pad behind the popliteal space.
5. Install the thigh pad.
6. Install the tibial pad.
7. Align the horizontal axis of rotation.
8. Position the scapular pad.
9. Secure the chest pad.
10. Move the patient to anatomical zero.
11. Adjust the extension and flexion stops.

All positioning is marked for easy software input and for ease of reproducing the setup for future test and/or exercise.

The Torso Rotation (TR) Testing and Rehabilitation Unit allows for identification of muscular strength and ROM deficits along with strengthening of back and abdominal muscles in a functional rotational pattern (Fig. 4.5). The patient is seated in a hip and knee flexed position of 90 degrees. The patient's rotational axis is aligned with the unit by a motorized vertically adjustable seat and horizontally adjustable seat back. The upper body is centered by the curved chest pad. The TR stabilization system for the lower body incorporates foot-bindings on the footplates to prevent leg motion and a lap belt which restricts fore/aft or up/down pelvis movement.

The following steps are required for mechanical setup:

1. Have the patient assume an upright seated position on the seat.
2. Adjust the seat height.
3. Adjust the footplate height.
4. Align the patient axis.
5. Tightly secure the lap belt.
6. Secure the lateral pelvic stabilization pads.
7. Install the knee pad assembly.
8. Secure the chest pad.
9. Move the patient to machine zero.
10. Set the range motion stops.

Lifting Capability Screening and Training System

The LIFTASK Lifting Capability Screening and Training System has been designed to screen individuals for functional deficits that may increase their risk of sustaining a back injury. This device enables simulation of specific lifting tasks. In addition to pre-employment and preplacement screening, the LIFTASK system can be used in the late stages of rehabilitation or to educate workers/athletes in efficient lifting techniques or simply for a work hardening program (Fig. 4.6).

Designed with a removable handle for custom-designed task simulation, the LIFTASK system allows lifting from the platform to 80 inches overhead and 30 de-

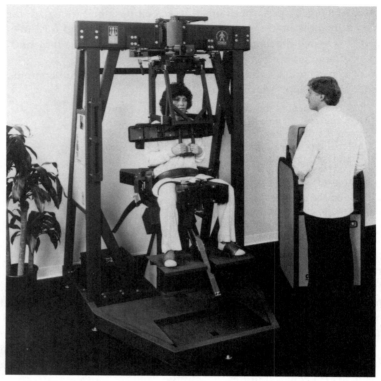

Figure 4.5. Cybex Torso Rotation Testing and Rehabilitation Unit (TR). Photograph courtesy of Cybex.

grees off the vertical axis. A variable position shelf allows simulation of lifts with a starting point other than the platform while a foot-placement grid ensures reproducibility of positioning.

The basic mechanical principles of the back testing dynamometers are consistent with all present and past systems. The dynamometer contains the same servosystem control for isokinetics throughout the range. This means that the same input/ output relationships are held to allow for the same basic measurement concepts. The back systems do have a greater force measurement capacity than the extremity unit (440 ft-lb for TEF and TR and 500 lb for LIFTASK).

The back systems were the first of the Cybex computer-enhanced systems that give immediate real-time displays on the screen along with processed data for measurements such as work, power, and endurance/fatigue. Protocols consisting of varied speeds, repetitions, and rest periods may be automatically controlled from the clinical work station (CWS) or may be operated manually by the use of the computer override.

All measurements are accurate and reliable (23). The repeatability of even the prototype TEF and TR was extremely high for both reproducibility and test-retest repeatability (23). Correlation coefficients for torque production on TEF resulted in r values greater than 0.91 and on TR resulted in r values greater than 0.96 for men and 0.90 for women.

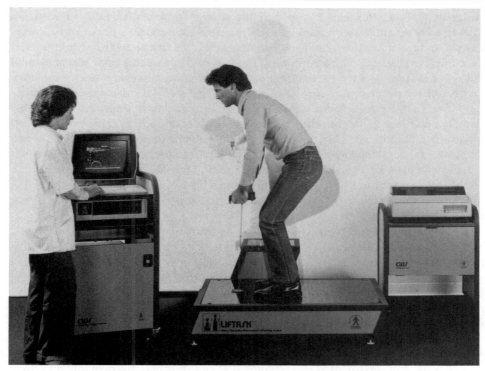

Figure 4.6. Liftask Lifting Capability Screening and Training System. Photograph courtesy of Cybex.

The basic components of the computer system are the graphics monitor (green display), disk drive unit (Cybex operating system, two 640kb floppy disk drives using 5¼-inch double-sided, quad-density diskettes) and keyboard (full-featured with numeric keyboard and several special function keys). This is on a single cart with a tiltable monitor holder and lower, upper keyboard shelves to allow for operation in a sitting or standing position.

Electronically interfaced is the speed controller and color graphics printer. The controller automatically sets the speed of the system dynamometers to the speed you indicate in the software (0 to 180 degrees/second on TEF and TR; 36 inches/second on LIFTASK). The multicolor graphics printer (black, blue, red, violet, brown, and orange) enables the clinician to maintain a hard copy of clinical records in numeric and graphic format. The printer is reliable, relatively quiet, and moderately slow for graphic reports with moderate speed for numeric reports.

In general, the CWS has the advantages and drawbacks of the simplicity and complications of a floppy disk system. The CWS is dedicated to the operation of the system, collecting and reporting data; it does not run other software.

The software package for back systems has all the basic features as described in the 340 extremity system. The main menu operations consist of Patient Information, Test/Exercise Mode, Display/Print Reports, Create/Update Protocols, and Calibration. All sections are extremely inclusive, especially the Clinical History section. Basic or detailed information may be typed in and stored. Basic and valuable information such as body weight is used to compute automatically the patient's peak torque (force) as a percentage of body weight. The clinical history is the first step toward computerizing clinical evaluation, with key prompts for a clinical or research tool. Mechanism of injury, predisposing activity/condition, onset of symptoms, previous back problems, number of recurrences, and time of recovery are just some of the categories listed.

The Test/Exercise Mode allows the clinician to perform a test or exercise session. The software guides the clinician through patient setup, trial repetitions (in Test Mode only), and the actual test or exercise. The system provides both tones and monitor display for combined audiovisual feedback. For example, the TEF computer issues a single tone to signal the beginning of a set, a second tone to seek the extension stop, a double-pitched tone to start the repetitions, and a high-pitched tone signals the end of each set. At the conclusion of a test session, there is also the option of redisplaying the data gathered by the system.

The Display/Print reports mode also has some advantages and disadvantages. The real-time graphic curves displayed during a test or exercise session may be displayed on the monitor screen only at the time of test or exercise and cannot be stored or printed in the present configuration. The curves that are stored from the real-time date are the maximum points curve, average points curve, and a single real-time curve (the best work repetition). It is recommended that data for each patient be stored on its own floppy disk. Each patient disk can store up to 50 tests.

Following a test, the CWS software immediately calculates peak torque (force), angle (height) of peak, peak torque (force) percent of body weight, acceleration time, time to peak, torque (force) at two additional angles (heights), average force, average power, total work, and maximum range of motion. Torque (force), work and power ratios for each speed are also calculated for Trunk Flexion/Extension and Torso Right Rotation/Left Rotation. These data can be displayed and/or printed in both numeric and graphic form even while other patients are being tested or exercised. While the real-time curves can only be redisplayed during the Test Validation Routine following a test session, the numeric and graphic reports can be produced at any time with the reports module. Reports printed consist of initial, status, progress, and discharge reports. The format selected under graphic and/or numeric may be Torque vs Position, Peak/Max Torque vs Speeds, Average Power vs Speeds, and Endurance/Fatigue.

Calibration and calibration verification of each of the units and system are as described in the section on the 340 system.

A full back testing system, consisting of TEF, TR, and LIFTASK, which includes three CWSs and two printers, occupies a minimum floorspace of 11 ft × 20 ft.

Clinically, the prototype Cybex back systems were utilized in the objective assessment and treatment of patients with chronic back pain with excellent results (24). Normative data collection was also undertaken for studies on the quantification of lumbar function (22, 23, 25–27).

Clinical results of the TEF unit (production model) have recently been described on a varied caseload. Timm (28) described the evaluation, treatment, and progress of one patient who had triple spinal surgery and one patient who had had a cerebrovascular accident. In both cases, Timm found that the TEF was an efficient and effective tool.

Advantages and Disadvantages

A number of clinicians were contacted regarding what they like and dislike about the Cybex system, the Cybex II or II+ system.

Advantages

1. Cybex users are dealing with a known quantity as these systems have been in use for a number of years. They also feel that physicians are familiar and comfortable with the information provided by this system.

2. Users indicate that they feel they are dealing with an established company that has developed service capabilities which meet their needs at least adequately. Users also indicate that they feel that the company has a representative system that enables them to be aware of product changes and general information.

3. The Cybex system is known for its safety because it is a passive system. This strength was cited by many users.

4. The flexibility enabling the use of this equipment over multiple joints and patterns was viewed as a significant strength by most users.

5. Cybex is a computer-enhanced rather than computer-controlled system; this allows a manual mode of exercise and was cited as a strength by many users. Thus even if the computer was malfunctioning an individual could still use the system; the system would not be shutdown by computer or disk/software problems.

Disadvantages

1. Cybex II or II+ does not have computer storage capabilities. This is a significant problem which limits the retrieval of information. (The new 340 system supposedly corrects this problem.)

2. As a passive system, 300 degrees/second may be a bit slow. This is particularly true in clinics using the equipment for upper extremity exercise.

3. Clinicians indicate that the noise generated by the system is distracting to some centers. (The 340 system supposedly corrects/diminishes this problem.)

4. Many users feel that the requirement of space and the numerous parts required to make the Cybex system flexible are also problematic. Users indicate that it is still somewhat difficult to get the right adapters in their hands at the correct moments.

5. Because the Cybex is a passive system, it does not allow the testing or the rehabilitation of eccentric muscle components.

Summary

The Cybex systems were the first isokinetic machines available for clinical use. They have been proven to be clinically dependable and provide an excellent tool for rehabilitation and exercise. The passive nature of the system allows only concentric contraction. Rather than present numerous case studies on equipment use, readers are urged to peruse the provided references.

REFERENCES

1. Axtell RS, Gravenstein RO, Lanese RR: The relationship between peak and mean torque in isokinetic exercise (abstract). *Med Sci Sports* 1986; 18:56
2. Flagge KF, Baker LR: Reliability of an isokinetic power—endurance test on femoris (abstract). *Phys Ther* 1986; 66:803
3. Francis K, Hoobler T: Comparison of peak torque values of the knee flexor and extensor muscle groups using the Cybex II and the Lido 2.0 isokinetic dynamometers (abstract). *Phys Ther* 1986; 66:809
4. Halbach JW, Davies GJ, Gould JA, et al: Relationship between torque acceleration energy and average power of the quadriceps and hamstrings determined by computerized Cybex testing (abstract). *Med Sci Sports Exerc* 1983; 15:144
5. Johnson J, Siegel D: Reliability of an isokinetic movement of the knee extensors. *Res Q* 1978; 49:88–90
6. Kozlowski BA: Reliability of isokinetic torque generation in chronic hemiplegic subjects (abstract). *Phys Ther* 1984; 64:714
7. Little KD, Sinning WE: Reliability of maximal isokinetic strength and work measures (abstract). *Med Sci Sports Exerc* 1985; 17:247
8. Moroz JS, Sale DG: Evaluations of the torque transducer of the Cybex II dynamometer (abstract). *Med Sci Sports Exerc* 1985; 17:247
9. Murray, DA, Harrison E, Wood GA: Cybex II reliability and validity: An appraisal (abstract). *Med Sci Sports Exerc* 1982; 14:153
10. Nielson DH, Hellwig EV, Swanson KL, et al: Measurement reliability of isokinetic strength (abstract). *Phys Ther* 1986; 66:804
11. Timm KE: Validation of the Johnson anti-shear accessory as an accurate and effective clinical isokinetic instrument. *J Orthop Sports Phys Ther* 1986; 7:298–303
12. Davies GJ: *A Compendium of Isokinetics in Clinical Usage*, La Crosse, WI: S and S Publishers, 1984
13. Fink MA, Bloecher J, Collins DT, et al: The effects of varying speeds of isokinetic exercise on physiological parameters and work output (abstract). *Phys Ther* 1985; 65:711
14. Knapik JJ, Jones BH, Bauman C, et al: Relationship between peak torque, average torque and total work in an isokinetic contraction (abstract). *Med Sci Sports Exerc* 1982; 14:178
15. Loving MH, Millsaps TK, Gossman, MR, et al: Relationship between muscle length and isokinetic torque and power in healthy males and females with "loose" and "tight" hamstrings (abstract). *Phys Ther* 1985; 65:700
16. Manning JM, Dooly-Manning C: Anaerobic power tests which can be used interchangeably (abstract). *Med Sci Sports Exerc* 1986; 18:24–25
17. Romanello ML: Torque acceleration energy, total work capacity, power, and endurance in the hamstring and quadricep muscle groups (abstract). *Phys Ther* 1985; 65:733
18. Sapega AA, Drillings G: The definition and assessment of muscular power. *J Orthop Sports Phys Ther* 1983; 5:7–9
19. Schlinkman B: Norms for high school football players derived from Cybex Data Reduction Computer. *J Orthop Sports Phys Ther* 1984; 5:243–245
20. Sherman WM, Armstrong LE, Murray TM, et al: Recovery of muscular strength, power and work capacity following intense endurance exercise: The marathon (abstract). *Med Sci Sports Exerc* 1982; 14:135
21. Siewart MW, Davies GJ, Ariki PK, et al: The effects of short arc terminal extension isokinetic exercise on the torque acceleration energy of the quadriceps (abstract). *Phys Ther* 1985; 64:732
22. Thompson NN, Gould JA, Davies GJ, et al: Descriptive measures of isokinetic trunk testing. *J Orthop Sports Phys Ther* 1985; 7:43–49
23. Smith SS, Mayer TG, Gatchel RJ, et al: Quantification of lumbar function: 1. Isometric and multi-speed isokinetic trunk strength measures in sagittal and axial planes in normal subjects. *Spine* 1985; 10:757–764
24. Mayer TG, Gatchel RJ, Kishino N, et al: Objective assessment of spine function following industrial injury: A prospective study with comparison group and one-year follow-up. *Spine* 1985; 10:482–493
25. Kishino ND, Mayer TG, Gatchel RJ: Quantification of lumbar function: 4. Isometric and isokinetic lifting simulation in normal subjects and low-back dysfunction patients. *Spine* 1985; 10:921–927

26. Mayer TG, Smith SS, Keeley J, et al: Quantification of lumbar function: 2. Sagittal plane trunk strength in chronic low-back pain patients. *Spine* 1985; 10:765-772

27. Mayer TG, Smith SS, Kondraske G, et al: Quantification of lumbar function: 3. Preliminary data on isokinetic torso rotation testing with myoelectric spectral analysis in normal and low-back pain subjects. *Spine* 1985; 10:912-920

28. Timm KE: Case studies: Use of the Cybex trunk extension flexion unit in the rehabilitation of back patients. *J Orthop Sports Phys Ther* 1987; 8:578-581

5

Kin-Com System

The Kin-Com was the first active system available in the United States. The system was developed and marketed in Canada and distributed to the United States through the Chattecx Corporation, a subsidiary of the Chattanooga Corporation.

The Kin-Com functions through a computer-controlled feedback system. Three primary signals are monitored and controlled (force, angle, and velocity). The computer is able to control or adjust the velocity or force according to the feedback it receives from the actuator. The force signal is generated in the load cell which serves as the input to the system from the actuator. The velocity signal is generated via a tachometer within the dynamometer head, and the angle signal is generated through a mechanical system, also within the dynamometer head.

The force and velocity are controlled through a hydraulic system within the Kin-Com. Specifically, a computer signal opens or closes the servovalve between the pump and the actuator to control force and velocity. This function is performed 100 times per second to maintain appropriate control of movement.

Because the system is computer controlled, it is dependent upon both software and hardware for function. It has now been available for several years and has gone through several major software updates and mechanical modifications. As the system has developed, the introduction of an upper extremity chair, trunk testing adapter, and electromyogram (EMG) system has enhanced its clinical and research potential.

The system's software controls both the exercise modes and the data acquisition and storage. The software enables a variety of parameters to be displayed and printed. All data can be stored on the computer's hard disk so that the comparison of a patient's strength performance from one visit to the next is possible. In addition, specific training protocols for an individual can be written and stored for easy access at each clinic visit. A strong feature of the system is its ability to correct for gravity and thus give all information in a gravity-corrected format.

The reliability of the system has been demonstrated by independent reviewers and it has been shown to be extremely accurate.

Specifications

The Kin-Com functions off a hard-drive IBM computer system. It controls velocity of movement through 210 degrees/second. An exciting option is the ability to set both minimum and maximum force limits during the velocity-controlled motion. Thus, the patient needs to generate a set minimum force in order to activate the movement, but must stay under the set maximum force to protect against unwanted joint stress.

Four models of exercise are available through the system. The isometric mode can be programmed to allow for multiple isometric contractions throughout a set range of motion. Again, a maximum force limit can be set to protect the joint. Graphic and numeric display on the computer's monitor during exercise can provide the patient with immediate feedback for motivation purposes.

A passive mode of exercise allows the Kin-Com to function as a continuous passive motion (CPM) device. The range of motion for this activity is computer controlled and therefore can be used to provide passive stretching. In addition, by setting a maximum force limit in the program, patients can apply a minimal force against the load cell without the machine shutting off. If this set force is exceeded, however, the machine will automatically shut off and any undesired maximal contractions can thus be avoided. In this way, submaximal training is also possible in this mode.

The isokinetic mode involves a constant velocity movement while the force production is variable. The Kin-Com "ramps" from initial force production to terminal velocity and then maintains the velocity at the preselected speed. This acceleration from 0 degrees/second to the preselected velocity can be set at low, medium, or high. Range of motion is programmed into the computer prior to the start of exercise by manually placing the limb in the desired "start" and "stop" positions. The exercise cycles can then be performed at different speeds and with different modes of contraction (i.e., passive, concentric, or eccentric). A minimum force required to initiate and maintain movement can be set by the therapist prior to exercise. This pre-loading option is designed to prevent unrestricted acceleration. Thus, the isokinetic mode controls velocity while force production varies.

The fourth mode of exercise available with the Kin-Com system is the "force mode." The isotonic or force mode is designed to control force while speed varies. This mode allows the patient to accelerate and decelerate the limb through his/her own muscular output. Once again, the clinician can establish a minimum force that the subject must exceed in order to accelerate the lever arm, an option that has important functional implications.

Within the force, isokinetic, and passive modes, clinicians can choose a variety of combinations of concentric, eccentric, and passive exercise. The concentric/concentric, eccentric/eccentric, concentric/eccentric, or eccentric/concentric exercise options can be used for training of agonist only or agonist/antagonist muscle groups.

The Kin-Com can be used for a variety of joints. A specific adapter for trunk testing and a special stabilization chair for upper extremity exercise are also available.

Data Collection

Data can be collected in either the evaluation or the training mode. Force data are provided in Newtons. Torque data can also be provided if the clinician measures the lever arm and feeds it into the computer prior to exercise. The data also can be corrected for gravity, thus allowing more accurate comparisons. In addition, EMG activity can be monitored simultaneously with force output through the use of a special EMG unit.

Data collected during the training mode is time based; data collected during the evaluation mode is angle or joint position based (Figs. 5.1 and 5.2).

Peak and average force data at any speed of contraction can be readily collected under the evaluation mode where there is a pause after each repetition. Data for any endurance type of exercise that requires multiple, continuous repetitions must be gathered under the training mode.

Under the evaluation mode, force data are automatically averaged over the number of repetitions completed for a given trial. The force curve is then displayed along with the average velocity and joint angle curves. The current software does not calculate power and work measurements, but will provide right/left comparisons, eccentric/concentric comparisons, flexion/extension ratios, etc. (Fig. 5.3). Under the training mode, peak and average force for each repetition must be gathered by the clinician from the time-based display on the monitor. Movement of the cursors around the repetition of interest will give the average force and peak force of that curve. That value can then be recorded by the clinician. This process must be repeated for each repetition of interest. All data collected under the evaluation or training modes can be stored for future reference.

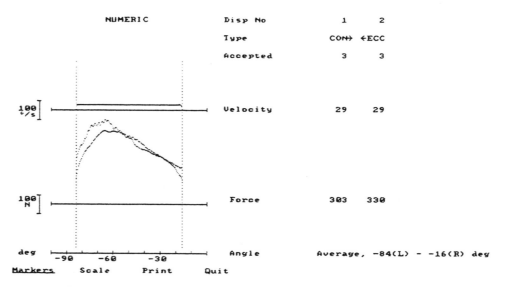

Figure 5.1. Example of force data display, collected under the evaluation mode.

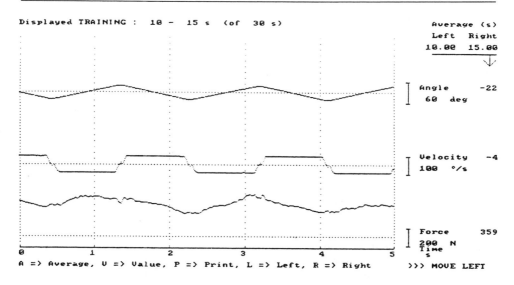

Figure 5.2. Example of force data displayed in time-based format, collected under training mode.

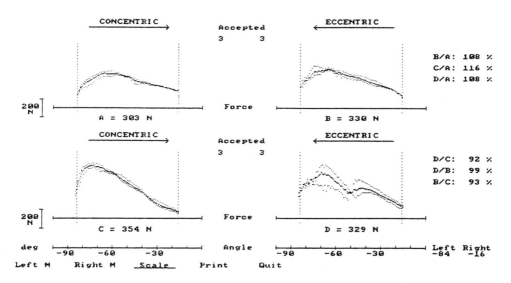

Figure 5.3. Example of force data display comparing one limb to the other and eccentric to concentric ratios (evaluation mode).

Clinical Applications

We frequently will begin using a passive mode of exercise early in the rehabilitation sequence. Patients are thus able to resist the movement within their pain tolerance and, at the same time, receive the benefits of the CPM movement. It is not uncommon for a person to be able to tolerate eccentric contractions prior to isotonic or isokinetic patterns. Eccentrics can be performed in a variety of exercise modes on this machine, but those performed under the passive mode may be more comfortable and easier for the patient to initiate. Thus, we frequently use the passive mode with eccentric contractions early in the rehabilitation process and then follow this with isometrics at multiple angles to allow facilitation of activity throughout the range of motion.

When a patient can tolerate multiple angle isometrics, a higher level of isometric force is requested and restricted range of motion isokinetics is begun. We again utilize eccentric as well as concentric forms of exercise in the isokinetic mode. As the patient begins to generate moderate levels of force, the "force mode" can be introduced. It is our opinion that the force mode allows a stronger neuromuscular integration and may be more functional in muscular demand. Because there may be a specificity of training relating to eccentric and concentric movements, both types of contraction should be used in training in order to stress the muscle's capability appropriately.

We frequently will use the passive mode between bouts of isokinetic and isotonic exercise to enable the patient's muscle to be "milked." This process allows a milking of metabolites and is relaxing to most patients.

We find the Kin-Com system to be applicable to research and clinical practice. It allows tremendous levels of force generation (approximately 2,000 Newtons) and provides excellent software, which not only controls the exercise programs but also collects and stores data. It is an excellent device for the setting involved with clinical and research efforts. Users agree that the Kin-Com is one of the best tools available for knee rehabilitation.

Advantages and Disadvantages

Advantages

1. Users feel that the Kin-Com has a stable platform and provides many exercise, data collection, and storage capabilities.

2. Multiple exercise modes are available including eccentric, concentric, isometric, and passive exercise. Users report that the multiple modes enable them to be flexible in individualizing treatment programs.

3. The new computer makes the Kin-Com more "user friendly," allowing greater independence of use by the clinician and patient alike. Users can also gain access to the system more easily and quickly.

4. Because of the tremendous torque capabilities, many users feel that this is the best available system for knee rehabilitation.

5. Users are comfortable knowing that the Chattanooga Corporation is the primary structure behind this product.

Disadvantages

1. Users find that it is somewhat difficult to interpret the printouts from the unit. It is often necessary to simplify the information in order to provide the physician with a more clinically meaningful report.

2. Some users indicated that they would like to exercise their patients at speeds greater than 210 degrees/second. The trade-off is that patients can generate greater torques within the available velocity spectrum.

3. Users report that some of the specific joint setups are awkward; this may be related to the stabilization and physical stature of the equipment.

4. One of the strengths but also weaknesses of the system is that it is computer controlled. The computer-controlled system is versatile and adaptable, but if there are problems related to either the software or hardware the system does not function.

5. The newest software does not measure work or power, data that many clinicians feel are important.

6

Lido System

Loredan Biomedical manufactures three different isokinetic dynamometry systems: the Lidoback, the Passive Multijoint System, and the Active Multijoint System. The Lidoback and the Passive Multijoint System use a hydraulic-based dynamometer, using a valve opening controlled by a microprocessor located within the dynamometer. The Active Multijoint System uses robotic technology to control the rotational component of the dynamometer, while measuring torque with strain gauges located within the axis. More complete descriptions of the specifics of each dynamometer are included below. All of the dynamometers are controlled by and resultant data reduced through use of software written for an IBM PC.

Passive Isokinetic Actuator

Inherent in the design of the passive actuator is that it may only move when an external torque is applied to its output shaft. Therefore, its use is limited to concentric exercise. (In fact, the force of gravity and inertial forces at high speeds may result in some eccentric exercise with a passive actuator.) Its principle of operation is hydraulic; a rotary actuator is used to move oil through a valve whose orifice size varies to control applied resistance. Measurement of position and torque is made by potentiometer and oil pressure transducers.

The actuator consists of a cylindrical volume divided into two chambers by a fixed and a movable vane. As the shaft rotates, oil is swept out of one chamber through a valve and into the other chamber. The valve opening is continuously varied by electrical means to provide a resistance producing a constant angular velocity.

The valve size is computed in a local microcomputer according to algorithms using set speed, position, torque, and shaft velocity as their inputs. The microcomputer and algorithms control valve opening through a combination of closed loop servo-control and a self-calibrating scheme based on automatic checks of its own performance.

The local microcomputer also allows control at the actuator through a panel which also keeps a running display of peak torque, in addition to handling serial communications between it and an IBM computer running the control, analysis, and storage program. Thus, a major advantage of the passive dynamometer is the ability to use it independent of the IBM PC.

The slowest speed that can be accurately tested on the passive dynamometer is 60 degrees/second on the multijoint unit and 30 degrees/second on the Lidoback unit. Clinicians who wish to test individuals at a slower velocity (i.e., isometrically) cannot accomplish this with a passive dynamometer-based system. Thus, this comprises a disadvantage in the passive dynamometer-based multijoint unit and the Lidoback.

Active Actuator

In distinction to the Loredan passive actuator, the active actuator, in an exercise or test mode, only moves when it moves itself. It is capable both of absorbing energy (when it emulates a passive actuator) and supplying energy to the exercising limb. Thus it is capable of being an exercise load for both concentric and eccentric exercise. Its principle of operation is control of motor speed according to a computer model of a physical system. Torque measurement is by strain gauges applied diagonally to the output shaft and position is by potentiometer.

The load consists of a high performance servomotor whose output speed is reduced by a gearless, lash-free mechanism designed for the robotics industry. Tachometer information is fed back to a high-gain servoamplifier resulting in accurate regulation of velocity.

The motor speed command is developed by a local microcomputer according to algorithms that model a rotating system with inertial and resistive components as well as a speed governor. Also available are isotonic models which are used to allow torque breakaway and eccentric exercise modes.

In distinction to the passive actuator control, this active process is only available by linkup with an IBM computer with matching software.

Because the actuator is capable of applying large amounts of force, elaborate, redundant safety systems and self-checks are a part of every actuator.

Safety Systems for the Active Lido

It is axiomatic that an exercise system capable of applying significant eccentric loads must have as its highest design priority the prevention of injury because of excessive loading. Operator error, innate or systematic flaws, and component breakdown are problems that must be prevented from transmitting abnormal loads to patients.

Each exercise mode and choice of joint contains important restrictions on operation designed to prevent injury. These include limits on range of motion, speeds, and torque. Attempts to exceed these limits when setting range limits will be unsuccessful. Eccentric torque is further limited to the peak torque of the previous concentric effort. This prevents the application of dangerously large eccentric loads while allowing heavy loads for muscles that are capable of handling them. Initial arm movements (i.e., positioning to set limits, doing a gravity compensation maneuver, certain other nonexercise arm movements) are operated at a minimum motor power level sufficient to complete the movements with all limbs likely to be encountered.

The first barrier to system breakdown is, of course, to build it to high standards of ruggedness and quality. The highest quality glass epoxy circuit boards, electronic components, and gold-plated connectors have been used throughout. In addition, the system itself must be designed so that the breakdown of any part does not produce an unacceptable movement of the exercise arm. The subsystems to be dealt with are torque, position and velocity measurement, the control elements, controller computer integrity, integrity of the serial link to the controlling IBM PC, and methods of shutting down the system in case of failure.

The controller compares its commands with all the measured conditions. In addition, the measurements are checked for consistency with each other. Measurements that are inconsistent with human physiology or machine capability are detected. Any inconsistency or troublesome condition is flagged, causing the system to shut itself down immediately. Because of the intelligent nature of these checks, it is virtually impossible for a control failure to go undetected. However, as a final backup, the patient may shut down the system with a button. It is typical of the failsafe philosophy used throughout the design of the system that breakage of the wires to the button will shut the system down.

The controlling computer performs internal checks on the integrity of its own subsystems. If this checks out, it performs a patterned behavior that is monitored by an entirely separate system. A failure of the computer is detected within $1/50$ of a second (.02 second), shutting the system down, using pathways entirely independent of those used by the computer.

If there is a failure of the IBM PC to communicate with the controller, the controller turns everything off and then locks itself up. The system is shutdown both by the computer and the system monitoring the computer.

As already mentioned, should a patient become alarmed, he/she may press a button that shuts down the system.

There are eight different methods of shutting down the system, exclusive of the power switch, all eight are independent, each adequate to bring the arm to a quick halt. These methods are distributed or shared among the computer, its monitor, and the patient button so that each has control of several methods of stopping the motor. A runaway system would require the simultaneous failure of eight rugged systems, each designed with a failsafe philosophy.

Each subsystem is designed so that a power failure will shut down the system. This extends to the external IBM PC. In fact, if the IBM PC should become disconnected from the system during any time the motor is on, the motor will be halted in a fashion requiring that the system be turned off and then turned on to resume operation. This is to ensure that operation is not possible without full-system integrity.

In summary, the best quality materials and construction techniques have been used to provide a high degree of reliability. Extensive internal safety and operational checks are made at a rate of speed ensuring nearly instantaneous response. Many redundant and failsafe pathways are utilized when stopping the motor. The integrity of the computer is checked by an independent, simple external system which utilizes its own separate pathways to shutdown the system. Every available technique has been used to produce an extremely safe system.

Gravity Compensation/Elimination

Accounting for the effect of gravity on isokinetic measures of muscle performance is well established in the literature. Accounting for the effect of gravity is available in all isokinetic systems manufactured by Loredan Biomedical Company; this is accomplished in two different ways. In the passive isokinetic actuators, the body segment is dropped through the desired excursion, and the resultant torque is recorded. Through software algorithms, this torque due to the weight of the segment is subtracted or added (as appropriate) to the torque recordings during the isokinetic bouts of exercise. Loredan refers to this as gravity compensation. In the active system, the segment is also allowed to drop through the desired excursion. Software algorithms then account for the weight of the limb and lever arm, resulting in the limb and lever arm of the dynamometer "floating freely" through space. Loredan refers to this as "gravity elimination."

The "gravity elimination" paradigm offers a unique advantage in its ability to assess the muscle performance in individuals with less than fair strength. By producing just enough assistance to the limb to compensate for the limb's weight, a subject will be able to produce concentrically or eccentrically a torque recording with the active actuator; the subject may not be able to do the same with the passive actuator.

Multijoint Setup

Both the active and passive multijoint units utilize the same basic clinical setup procedures. These include the use of the multijoint bench for positioning of the patient and the dynamometer (Fig. 6.1). In the position shown, the patient can be positioned supine or sidelying for testing of shoulder (all planes), hip (all planes), and ankle (sagittal plane). The bench has the capability of adjusting to become a chair for use with a knee setup (Fig. 6.2).

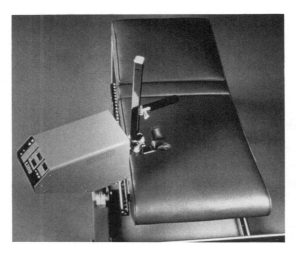

Figure 6.1. Multijoint bench.

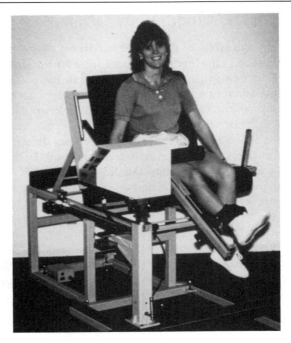

Figure 6.2. Multijoint system in knee flexion/extension position.

The dynamometer of both multijoint systems is mounted on a pedestal. The dynamometer is allowed rotational movement around the axis of the pedestal with lock-in points every 45 degrees around the axis (Fig. 6.3). The dynamometer can be raised or lowered using a crank located at the base of the pedestal. There is no adjustment to tip the dynamometer backward or forward. The pedestal is in turn mounted on a track system (Fig. 6.4), and using roller bearings, the dynamometer is allowed forward and backward as well as side to side motion of the dynamometer.

Attached to the sides of the bench are tracks that, through the use of keys, allow attachment of the dynamometer to the bench along the entire length of the bench (Fig. 6.5). This provides adjustment of superior-inferior positioning of the dynamometer relative to the patient.

Advantages and Disadvantages

Advantages

1. Space Considerations. The versatility of the bench and the tracking system to move the dynamometer eliminates the need of having multiple benches and chairs for different joint setups, thus providing an advantage for the clinician who has limited space in which to operate. This is, in fact, one of the major advantages offered by either of the Lido multijoint systems in that the entire system, including the IBM PC, requires a 6.5 × 3 ft area of space for the dynamometer, and a 2 × 2 ft area for the computer and peripherals.

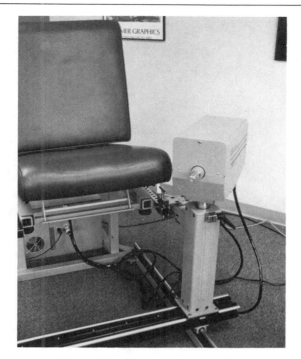

Figure 6.3.   Dynamometer rotation.

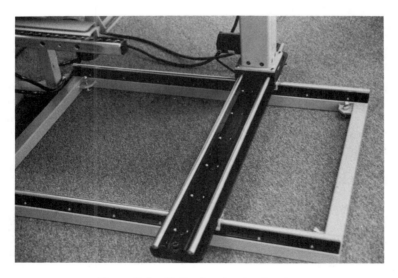

Figure 6.4.   Roller bearing tract system.

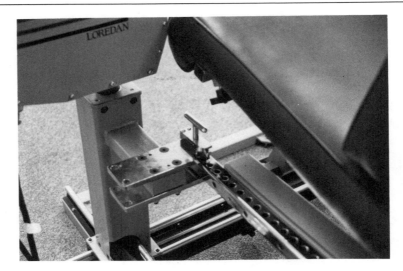

Figure 6.5. Lido track allowing dynamometer positioning.

2. Clinical Use. In performing bilateral testing, the dynamometer moves; the patient does not move. It is not necessary to move a patient when performing bilateral testing using either multijoint system, as the dynamometer is easily moved along the tracking system and attached to the other side of the bench. Thus, the assessment procedure is efficient and, in comparison with many other isokinetic systems, fast.

3. Serviceability. The dynamometer is attached to the pedestal with four bolts, all within easy access. Thus, if service to the dynamometer is necessary, the dynamometer is easily removed from the pedestal.

4. Support. The IBM PC, all peripherals and software (including one year of free updates) are included in the purchase price of each system.

Disadvantages

1. Accessibility. In the knee setup, the seat of the bench is higher than seat height. Thus, accessibility becomes a problem for small children and disabled individuals. This can also become a problem for a clinician working without supportive help to assist in transfers and who intends to use the dynamometer on disabled individuals or small children.

Lidoback

The Lidoback system (Fig. 6.6) allows isokinetic trunk testing in the sagittal plane only with the subject either in a standing (Fig. 6.7A) or sitting position (Fig. 6.7B). Adjustments of platform and seat height and roll pad position, are accomplished by the clinician by pushing buttons that control motors, and the relative positions of the adjustments are presented on a digital display (Fig. 6.8). Recording of these positions after the subject's position has been set becomes invaluable during

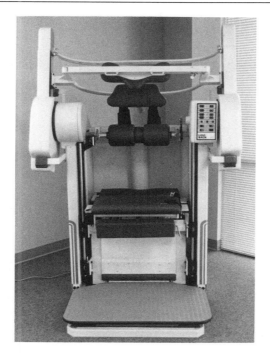

Figure 6.6. Lidoback system, an independent unit.

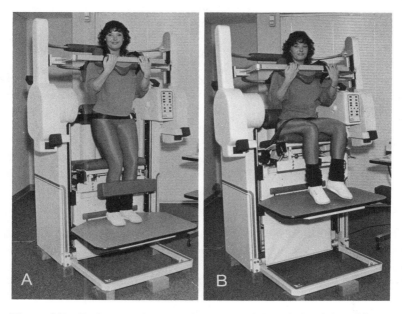

Figure 6.7. Patient can be tested in standing (A) or sitting (B) position.

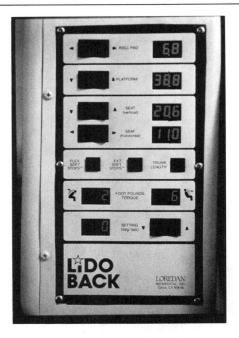

Figure 6.8. Digital display of adjustable parameters.

subsequent testing of the same individual in that position of testing can be accurately duplicated, thus improving test-retest reliability. The Lidoback occupies a 3 × 4 ft area, with a 2 × 2 ft area for the computer and peripherals.

Advantages and Disadvantages of Lidoback

As stated above, the Lidoback has the capability of testing individuals in either a standing or a sitting position. This versatility may be of importance for clinicians interested in using both test positions. Stabilization through the use of belts is adequate. At this time, the Lidoback does not provide the capability to test the trunk in other than sagittal plane motion. This is a disadvantage to clinicians who wish to test rotational trunk muscle performance. The Lidoback is quite large, and most components are not readily accessible. When servicing becomes necessary, this may present a problem.

Software for the Lidoback

The software for the Lidoback and the multijoint systems operate from the same basic menu (Fig. 6.9). The menu is designed in such a way that the usual assessment will begin using selection 1 first, selection 2 second, and so on. This may not necessarily be the case all the time, however. For example, in treating a patient who has been seen previously, a clinician may begin with selection 3 or 4. The software easily allows this. The menu is comprised of the following:

1. Patient Data Description

This is where the therapist enters the subject's name, age, height, weight, physician's name, etc. This information is used both in the descriptive portion of the report as well as in the calculation of some of the data (i.e., weight used in calculation of peak torque to body weight ratio).

2. Setup Test Parameters

This is where the clinician chooses different setup parameters to be used with each subject. With the active and passive multijoint systems, the choices include selection of joint to be tested, selection of plane to be tested, and selection of the speeds to be tested. In addition, the active multijoint system allows the clinician to choose at this time what type of contraction will be asked for, including concentric, eccentric, or continuous passive motion. In the concentric mode, the dynamometer is used in fashion identical with that used in the passive dynamometer. In the concentric-eccentric mode, the subject will concentrically push the limb in one direction, and at end of the excursion, the dynamometer will push against the limb to return to the starting position, with resistance offered by the subject through eccentric contraction of the desired muscle. In the continuous passive motion mode, the limb is moved back and forth through a set excursion, and the subject can either assist the dynamometer concentrically or resist it eccentrically during the exercise. As a safety precaution, in all exercise using the active dynamometer, upper limits of torque not to be exceeded can be set initially.

In the Lidoback software, the only choices the clinician needs to make in this menu selection are whether to test sitting or standing, and what speeds (up to maximum of 4) will be tested.

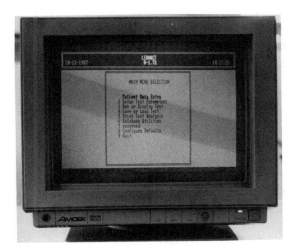

Figure 6.9. Basic menu of the Lido system.

3. Run or Display Test (Patient Data Collection)

This section has two modes. In the initial portion, the clinician must first select the extremity side (except Lidoback) and the speed to be tested. Once this is selected, the display is changed to a biofeedback mode. In this mode, the IBM PC is linked directly to the dynamometer's torque and position angle transducers, and the display on the screen includes pistons of two different colors whose amplitude is reflective of the amount of torque that the dynamometer is registering. This is real-time feedback and can be used by an exercising subject as objective biofeedback information concerning his/her performance.

It is in this mode that the clinician can begin collecting data. This is done by simply hitting the return key to begin collection and hitting the return key again to end collection of data.

Once data are collected, the software again enters the initial mode of the patient data collection section. Here, the collected data can be displayed in both a time-based fashion, as in a strip chart recording (Fig. 6.10) or a position-based display, with torque overlaps, as in Figure 6.11. The following measures are calculated:

1. *Peak Torque, the highest point on the torque curve.* If more than one repetition is displayed, then the highest peak torque is displayed. The units are foot-pounds.
2. *Average Peak Torque, the average of all the individual torque curve's peak torque.* The units are foot-pounds.
3. *Range of Motion,* the average range of motion (in degrees) accomplished over the number of repetitions displayed.
4. *Average work,* angular work is torque multiplied by the angular distance traversed. Thus, work is determined by calculating the area under the torque curve using the position trace as the x-axis. The average work is the total work done divided by the number of repetitions; the units are foot-pounds.

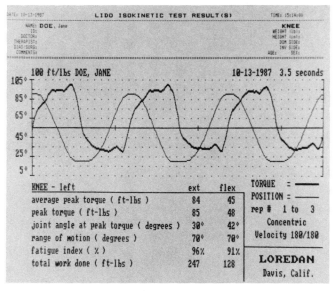

Figure 6.10. Strip chart recording of time-based data.

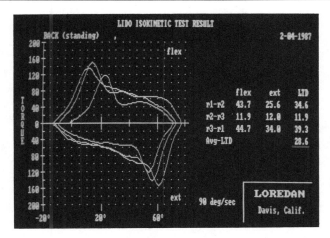

Figure 6.11. Position-based display of torque values.

5. *Fatigue Index.* This is a work-based measure. Each repetition's work value (y-axis) is plotted against repetition number (x-axis), and a linear regression is calculated. The predicted value of the last repetition is then expressed as a percentage of the predicted value of the first repetition. This percentage comprises the fatigue index. Thus, a 100% fatigue index indicates there is no torque decline over repetitions.

6. *Lido Confidence Value, or "LCV."* This value is calculated only in the position-based display; it is based on the total area of the subsequent torque curves that fall outside the initial torque curve, and it is then divided by the total work done in the initial torque curve. This number represents angular work of subsequent torque curves that is not in agreement with the initial torque curve; it is purported to be reflective of submaximal efforts on the part of the subjects, i.e., the greater the "LCV," the more likely the subject is performing at submaximal capacity. This is based on the notion that submaximal efforts are not likely to be reproducible. Although an intriguing idea, the validity of the "LCV" has yet to be determined.

4. Save or Load Test (Store/Retrieve Patient Data)

All patient data can be stored to floppy disks. The default is to store to the B drive of the IBM PC. Similarly, data can be retrieved from floppy disks. In retrieving data, a clinician is offered the choice of "patient parameters only" or "entire test." The former allows the clinician to recall only patient parameters (menu selection #1) of previous tests for use with follow-up testing; the latter loads all information, including data collected, from a previous test.

5. Print Test Analysis

The printout of an isokinetic assessment is shown in Figure 6.12. Calculation of all data is exactly the same as previously described in section #3/Run or Display Test data section of the menu. In addition, patient information is printed at the top of the printout.

6. Database Utilities

Progress reports can be printed from this section of the menu.

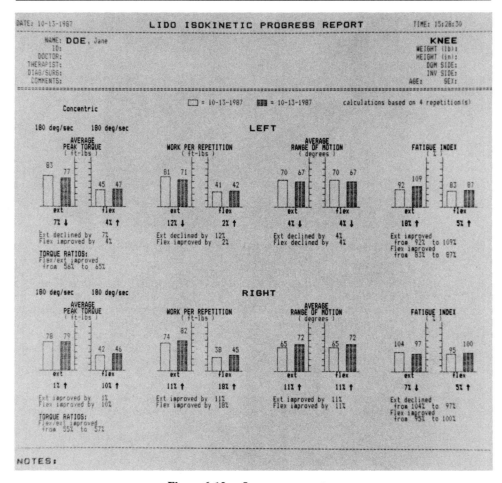

Figure 6.12. Summary report.

Advantages and Disadvantages of Software

This software is user friendly. The menu is clearly and logically structured, and all possible selections are conveniently displayed on the screen at all times. If you are uncertain, pressing the "escape" key on the IBM PC keyboard will nearly always return you to the previous menu selection. Even those who are unaccustomed to computers should find interaction with this software fairly comfortable. The biofeedback mode is both convenient and useful for subjects using the dynamometer as an exercise device. Displays of data from the data collection mode are flexible with regard to portions of the bout displayed; data can easily be printed using the print screen command of the IBM PC. Printouts supplied by the software are concise and include most of the useful information of an isokinetic assessment.

A disadvantage of the software is the inability to "window" the torque curves. If data collection within a specified arc of motion could be predetermined, then clinicians would be assured of making comparisons between tests of muscle performance based on similar conditions between tests. For example, in comparing an initial to a subsequent test, a clinician may note that a higher work value can be obtained during a second test for a particular patient. This higher value could be due to (1) a desired training effect or (2) the fact that the patient went through a larger excursion on the second test. At present, there is no way to control for this. By the same token, when soft-stops are used, peak torque will often occur when the dynamometer slows the limb down at the soft stop. Without the capability of "windowing" out the point in the range of motion where the soft-stop occurs, the peak torque at the soft-stop will be the peak torque recorded by the software on the printout.

Clinical Application

The Lido multijoint systems utilize a sliding-cuff to anchor the patient's limb to the dynamometer arm. This allows the system to adapt to changing components and not apply abnormal compressive loads to the rotating joint's articular surfaces.

The passive system is similar in application to the previously described isokinetic systems but does not offer speeds below 60 degrees/second. The active system allows the integration of passive motion and eccentric and concentric isokinetic exercises. The aforementioned special feature of gravity elimination provides the clinician the opportunity to record very low torque outputs from patients demonstrating greatly decreased strength levels. The myriad of combinations allowed by the active system gives great flexibility to the clinician in implementing a variety of rehabilitation protocols.

Advantages and Disadvantages

Advantages

1. Sliding-Cuff. This feature makes this system one of the most comfortable for patients. This feature allows the system to feel extremely smooth and comfortable.

2. Software Applications. These provide relevant information in an easily digested form.

3. Biofeedback/Visual Display. This provides excellent patient motivation.

4. Space Requirement. In many clinics, the limited space requirements are greatly appreciated.

Disadvantages

1. Low speed/isometric limitation of the passive system and the lack of eccentrics in the passive system are negative features.

2. The eccentric limitations, which are based on a concentric contraction, may not be the most applicable method of providing this limitation. Clinicians would like to be able to dial in their own limitations rather than base limitations on a concentric contraction which may not be reflective of eccentric ability.

3. Computer software and hardware safety features are required; however,

these have sometimes caused the system to shutdown, apparently without reason. Their sensitivity may need to be improved.

4. The bench is a bit high and some clinicians would like to see a better method of getting patients onto the bench. The height is uncomfortable for many.

Acknowledgment. The author thanks Phil Dempster of Loredan Biomedical Co. for assistance in the technical description of the dynamometers.

7

MERAC System

Today, there is an increasing number of individuals seeking medical aid and attention for complaints of the musculoskeletal (locomotor) system. Muscular-skeletal disorders comprise the greatest single cause of time loss, sick leave, and financial burden in the American work force. The magnitude of the socioeconomic effects of musculoskeletal dysfunction are undoubtedly greater than any one statistic.

Research and studies in the treatment of musculoskeletal dysfunction prove clearly that there is a greater need for effective treatment through improved diagnostic measures and treatment procedures. Improved techniques that involve basic therapeutic philosophies are needed as well as techniques applied to the preventive aspects of physical (musculoskeletal) conditioning programs. Prolonged dysfunction dramatically affects the musculoskeletal system and is complicated by soft tissue changes which in many cases become irreversible.

Proper treatment of body tissue and associated joints is a key in preventing irreversible and chronic dysfunction of the human system. There is an increased need for physical activity and our ability to screen and provide comprehensive clarifying examinations will play a major role in preventing the kinds of dysfunction that our patients experience through essential and nonessential physical activity.

History confirms the origins of exercise and there is ample evidence to demonstrate the importance of exercise. Strength training, dance, games, and more formal programs may be categorized as a general or specific exercise mode. Specific strengthening and strength testing may or may not diminish musculoskeletal dysfunction in the locomotor system.

The person involved in rehabilitation and training may abuse the musculoskeletal system through improper stretching, too much resistance, and/or poor biomechanics. Physical activities such as aerobic dance, jazzercise, and distance running may be hazardous and damaging formats for the deconditioned individual.

Some of the testing and treatment protocols used today are faulty due to lack of knowledge, and some of the individuals using these protocols lack the skill necessary to test and treat the "normal and abnormal" structures of the human system.

The role of the therapist, trainer, and other health clinicians is not just to understand and treat, but to guide and teach the patient to understand the musculoskeletal system through principles of bodily tolerance, constrained movements, duration of stress, joint function, and restoration of "balance."

The MERAC (Musculoskeletal Evaluation Rehabilitation and Conditioning) system is not only a testing musculoskeletal evaluative and rehabilitative machine, but it is a dynamic system allowing for several modes of exercise to be incorporated based on musculoskeletal dysfunction, pathology, and individual differences. It allows for exercise based on medical diagnosis and musculoskeletal tolerances and associated individual differences.

Proficiency in detecting and treating muscular pathology is gained through experience, repeated examination, and a thorough understanding of biomechanics. Treatment and testing protocols should provide a positive pain-free experience for the participant and the result should be improvement in function.

MERAC allows for the restoration of muscular movement patterns (physiologic training) and provides functional and qualitative measurements by which treatment and training can be objectively analyzed.

In any form of exercise, a muscle must have neurovascular function. Movements should be free of pain and circulatory disturbance. The function should be physiologic. Overuse and overstress in training and testing can lead to injury and have a catabolic effect.

Muscular skeletal "balance" is the optimal goal of rehabilitation. Testing and training systems should allow for "normal range of movement" without unnecessary stress to associated tissues, including ligaments, joint capsules, joint surfaces, and, more importantly, intra-articular structures.

The MERAC system, designed and manufactured by Universal, provides the clinician with the flexibility to treat the acute and chronic pathologic dysfunctions seen in American rehabilitation and conditioning settings today.

In developing a system for testing as well as strengthening and conditioning, Universal has taken into consideration safety and physiologic principles that provide low speed testing as well as maximum high-speed testing and isokinetic training. Stability and comfort are provided in isometrics and with individual dynamic variable resistive training. MERAC incorporates subsequent self-designed protocols to be incorporated in each exercise mode (isometric, isotonic, and isokinetic exercise). Testing procedures allow the clinician to work within safe and pain-free joint motion with varying therapeutic approaches depending on the participant's mental, physiologic, and anatomical capability. All strengthening exercise modes incorporate safety in treatment and testing adaptability of joint function; they also provide access to qualitative measurement in all parameters of exercise.

MERAC allows physiologic consideration of optimal speed resistance and duration of force and provides for optimal results, thus a complete and valid test.

Health clinicians who administer and provide therapeutic testing and training today look to the system that is economically attainable, is mechanically durable and stable, and provides exercise modes for a variety of pathologies and personal needs.

In summary, the MERAC system (1) incorporates physiologic movement patterns, and (2) incorporates physiologic and anatomical joint function through strengthening protocols, providing locking and stability techniques to be selective and specific in active participation in isometric, isotonic, and isokinetic exercise modes.

The MERAC system provides a realistic representation of physiologic and anatomical movements through its recording and software system and provides flexibility through its single-station system without instability via its "high tech" design. It ensures a more complete clinical examination and accurate diagnosis, and it provides procedures and therapeutic techniques that have not been available in our health care delivery system until now.

The existing philosophies of strength training incorporate concepts and beliefs from the earliest authors to modern-day contributors. Strengthening principles outlined a simple statement of providing a progressive degree of resistance to principles that exceed the highest limits of physiologic motor capability. We know the importance of contracting a muscle to the limits of its physiologic capacity in order to develop strength as well as power. Strength concepts involve static, dynamic, and explosive parameters.

Today's methods of strengthening are isometric, isokinetic, or isotonic. The method depends upon what property of the contracting muscle is held constant during exercise.

The MERAC system offers all forms of concentric exercise and lends the clinician the capability of load intensity through variable resistance training, isometric training, and isokinetic training. Isotonic training methods continue to be developed, yet all programs provoke questions in the area of "optimum loading frequency" and "duration of loading" and leave the clinician with concerns about joint movement and soft tissue involvement.

Isokinetics

The isokinetic approach to muscle assessment and training is important but it is only one approach to muscle testing and training. It eliminates the patient/participant from comprehensive protocols that employ isometrics and individual dynamic variable resistance training.

In the past, the concepts of isokinetics have limited the participant and clinician to testing protocols of 300 degrees/second as the highest speed available. The MERAC system gives the opportunity to collect data based on speeds of 500 degrees/second.

Isokinetic testing using the MERAC system provides reliable valid and reproducible measurements and provides a system for strengthening muscular endurance, training, and power training. The isokinetic mode allows for a physiologic muscular response by providing accommodating resistance to a set speed and allows for testing and training the low velocities as well as high velocities.

Isokinetics was first introduced in the 1960s; it is not new to the science of kinetics and strengthening. The isokinetic systems available in today's market all provide the ability to exert force continuously against the body at a set constant velocity.

The isokinetic system constrains the motion of the body so that the path followed centers itself with joint center rotation that the muscular system induces, thereby allowing muscle to contract at a constant velocity. If the body cannot be accelerated, any imbalanced force exerted against it is resisted by an equal and opposite reaction force. This isokinetic system at its most highly designed and technical state cannot assume the physiologic occurrences through angular velocity and muscular shortening as seen in free physiologic motion. Thus, musculoskeletal function cannot be duplicated by a machine based on the simplest geometric reasons. Accommodating resistance training is an important component of the MERAC system.

Isometrics

Isometric training was not given substantial attention until the late 1940s when Hellebrandt made known his findings in the area of strength training. Hellebrandt's research along with that of Müller and others reaffirm the theory that maximal training effects were positive and strength improved even if contractions were brief and not maximal.

Today, we recognize that submaximal effort does indeed improve strength. Isometric training has many considerations based on tension, the frequency of repetition, and duration of contractions.

In summary, isometric strengthening is an effective, safe, and acceptable mode of exercise, and it does produce strength increases. However, isotonic exercise appears to be more effective and more widely used.

It is important to note that the most effective isokinetic program has not been unequivocally defined. Adjustments to duration of contraction and frequency of repetition and training sessions are the keys in meeting the needs of individual muscles in patients with different pathologies.

Testing and Training Protocols

Selecting or defining an absolute testing and/or training protocol may produce a major error for the clinician without taking into consideration individual differences and pathology.

The influence of testing and training may be affected by:

1. Additional exercise and treatment modalities
2. Education of the patient to testing and training
3. The type of exercise mode
4. The selective range of motion for the program
5. Level of subjective pain
6. Effusion, soft tissue tenderness, and additional tissue response testing

Individual assessment must be performed prior to each test and/or training protocol. Following this assessment, modifications may be necessary prior to performing the exercise. It is important that education be given daily and that both short-term and long-term goals be identified. Motion will be modified on a daily basis based on the patient's response to testing, and alterations in repetition, sets and exercise frequency must be constantly reevaluated. Maximal vs submaximal training must again be looked at on a daily or at least frequent basis to facilitate progress in a positive direction.

There is no standard protocol in isometric, isotonic, and isokinetic modes of exercise although individuals have established some guidelines in reference to time, repetition testing, resistance applied in testing speeds isokinetically as well as maximal vs submaximal efforts.

In selecting a test and/or treatment protocol, individualized guidelines must be established for (1) time of initial test, (2) retest frequency, and (3) establishment of goals in the parameters of strength, speed, power, and endurance.

Guidelines are needed for dealing with joint range of motion, frequency of exercise sessions, time training vs repetition training, and controls over additional training modalities and procedures.

With these considerations, the MERAC offers six exercise modes that allow the adaptability of each of these considerations in an individual program.

The MERAC system has superior stability and the ability to increase informative data and calculations. The system allows testing speeds to be increased higher than other equipment and offers dynametric testing in three other modes of exercise. Continued investigation with variable parameters and protocols are warranted until enough information has been collected to provide direction in establishing specific procedures in testing and/or training.

Validation Studies

The Exercise and Sport Research Institute at Arizona State University recently conducted two independent tests on the MERAC system.

The first test was conducted to examine the validity and repeatability of torque measurements being quantified by the MERAC system. Torque values were extracted from MERAC using standard software features of the system and were then compared with the actual torques applied to the system by known weight.

The results of the analysis indicated that the torque measurements obtained from MERAC showed little difference from the actual torque values (overall mean difference of 1.2%). The results also demonstrated that the torque measurements were highly repeatable on a day-to-day basis (difference no greater than 1 ft-lb). Based on the results of this test, it was concluded that the torque values quantified by MERAC were valid and reliable.

The second test was conducted to determine the validity of angular velocities of the MERAC system. Velocities of the MERAC system, as quantified by the system hardware and extracted from the graphic display of system output, were compared with similar measures quantified independently using high-speed cinematography. Results of the comparison demonstrated that the two sets of angular velocity data were nearly identical for all conditions tested. Based on these results, it was concluded that the angular velocity measures obtained from the MERAC system were valid.

Self-Monitors for Accuracy

MERAC is a closed-loop system, meaning that the dynamometer is continuously self-monitored. High-speed microprocessors allow MERAC to check torque 1,000 times per second speed up to 11,333 times per second, and position 32,400 times per second. If at any time a system calibration is off, MERAC automatically adjusts for accuracy.

Undampened Signal Produces Real Data

MERAC produces more than just a curve. Fifty or more undampened data points are collected to plot each degree point on the graph. All data displayed are actual so you can be sure the data are real; this increases the validity of your test.

Bench and Dynamometer Stability

MERAC is the most stable system on the market today. The bench is constructed of 2 × 4 inch and 2 × 2 inch steel tubing. The heavy-duty dynamometer has a $5/16$ inch wall × $3^3/8$ inch telescopic support post with rugged $1/2$ inch plated mounting brackets to ensure superior stability even when testing the most powerful athlete. Because the bench and dynamometer are stable, data collected are from musculoskeletal movement only.

Joint Isolation

Without proper patient stabilization, external influences that cause muscle action can produce inaccurate test data. MERAC's positive strapping and support systems ensure proper joint isolation at all joint planes and testing modes. So, data collected are from the movement of the affected joint only.

Gravity Calibration

MERAC automatically calibrates to eliminate biased data produced by gravitational influences in each testing and training procedure.

Summary

The needs of your patients and profession demand a screening, testing, and rehabilitation system that is as competent as current technology will allow. MERAC offers Isokinetic, Isokinetic Fatigue, Isotonic, Isotonic Fatigue, Isometric, and Individualized Dynamic Variable Resistance (IDVR) modes.

The MERAC system provides test data, graph recordings, and printed results, which provide advanced information in the areas of strength, speed, motion, work fatigue/endurance, power, and exertion.

In addition, an undampened signal from a self-monitoring system, stable bench and dynamometer, proper joint isolation, and gravity calibration ensure that the data MERAC produces are valid and reliable.

MERAC features:

1. Isokinetic, Isokinetic Fatigue, Isotonic, Isotonic Fatigue, Isometric, and IDVR testing and conditioning modes
2. Speed spectrum to 500 degrees/second, torque spectra to 500 ft-lb
3. Easily adjustable attachments for all planes and testing procedures for the knee, ankle, wrist, shoulder, hip, and elbow
4. Patient and extremity stabilization for proper joint and muscle isolation
5. Electronic range of motion stops
6. Digital goniometer
7. Automatic gravity calibration
8. Data taken from an undampened signal
9. Self-monitoring for accuracy

10. Automatic data calculations
11. Graph enlargements and reductions possible after testing
12. Multiple test, patient to patient and bilateral comparisons
13. Protocol setup and storage
14. Complete printed results
15. Complete data storage

Evaluation

The data MERAC provides allow assessment of functional capabilities, strength, motion, power, and fatigue. From these data, an individualized program to achieve optimal musculoskeletal balance and function can be developed. In addition to assisting in designing a comprehensive rehabilitative or conditioning program, MERAC aids in the detection and prevention of potential pathologies.

Rehabilitation

MERAC offers six modes of exercise and a variety of attachments for developing protocols. MERAC also offers immediate visual and auditory biofeedback. Performance and test results can be instantly viewed on the monitor and quickly and concisely reviewed by you and your patient.

By choosing the desired exercise mode, and establishing the desired parameters of speed, resistance, time, joint position, and range of motion, rehabilitative programs can be designed and stored for all pathologies of the musculoskeletal system.

Conditioning

MERAC is a humanistic control system that provides maximal/submaximal strength training and sensory motor integration, making it ideal for conditioning. Because the speed spectra goes up to 500 degrees/second, neuromuscular training and strengthening can be more closely coordinated with the arthrokinematics of the human system.

As in rehabilitation, biofeedback plays an integral roll in training. In addition to providing instant visual feedback, MERAC allows comparison of present data with previously recorded results. Positive reinforcement through recognition of progress and goal achievement becomes a motivating force in conditioning and training.

Advantages and Disadvantages

Advantages

1. A variety of modes of exercise are available and enable clinicians to individualize exercise programs in unique ways.

2. In comparison with other systems the MERAC has an ease of operation that is superior. Many patterns can be handled by the patient independently.

3. The system allows high torque values as well as high speeds. This is particularly appreciated in athletic populations.

4. This system seems to be the most stable exercise platform available.

5. Excellent patient feedback is presented during exercise providing biofeedback and serving as a motivational tool.

Disadvantages

1. As with all systems on the market, retrieval of information is slower than desired but has been facilitated to print reports in less than 1 minute.

2. Specific graphs provide numeric information beyond what has been available and may not be understood or utilized clinically by all clinicians.

3. Retrieval of specific information in the printed form provides a complicated picture because of the quantity of data presented and less than optimal graphic description.

4. The lack of eccentric capabilities may be a limiting factor for this system. Further research will indicate how appropriate or necessary eccentric testing will be.

8

Summary

It should be obvious that significantly improved isokinetic equipment is available for the clinician of today. The selection of an isokinetic device should involve more than cost. Too often clinicians procure equipment without realizing the additional required efforts for said equipment to be functional. Ideally, one individual therapist should become the isokinetic "expert" in each clinic that possesses such equipment. This person handles all communication with the manufacturers and their representatives, organizes in-service programs based on clinical applications, and is responsible for designing the testing protocols. Many years of clinical training have led to the following recommendations for new users of isokinetic equipment:

1. Do not become frustrated—things will get better!
2. Do the setups; do not just watch someone else do them.
3. Allow the "expert" to do the majority of testing. This person then trains via in-services the rest of the staff but continues to be available for questions and guidance.
4. Standardize the clinic protocol for testing each individual joint and stick with that protocol for at least one year.
5. Remember isokinetics involves intense work by major muscle groups surrounding the joint. Hence, appropriate warm-up and stretching is essential before and after exercise. Ice, compression, and elevation are commonly recommended after heavy workouts; the noninvolved extremity must always be tested first.
6. Read all material that arrives with the unit and post these materials so they are available while clinicians become familiar with the particular positions and setups required for testing.
7. Become well-acquainted with your sales representative; this individual represents an important resource.
8. Do not view this piece of equipment as the only answer but rather as one part of the whole. Rehabilitation must degenerate into exercise.
9. Develop pictures and label pieces of equipment so that you are able to use equipment quickly and easily. Familiarity does not breed contempt.
10. Develop a network of friends who have similar devices. User groups have been popularized with computers and are an effective way of sharing and gaining from the errors and mistakes of others as they will gain from yours.

An obvious question is, "What piece of equipment is best for a particular setting?" What may seem to be a fairly easy question is, in fact, extremely difficult to answer. For some clinics a passive system will satisfy requirements and enable a large staff to interact and gain information on a variety of patients. Other clinics will need an active device as their staff may be required to be involved in research projects in which a variety of contractions must be measured. It should be noted that definitive studies as to what we are measuring have not yet been performed. The measurement of strength is not a direct but rather an indirect process. Our measurements are through the skeletal system and require us to be aware of the limitations this poses. Rather than recommend a single device, the following synopsis is a piece-by-piece description of what many clinicians found to be the major strengths or weaknesses of the available devices.

Ariel Computerized Exercise System

The computer controlling system is efficient and does an excellent job of establishing comparisons, thus minimizing operator setup time. The system is flexible with many exercise modes available. Ease of use with little supervision is another important feature, and there is excellent feedback to the patient during and after exercise. In addition, data may be stored for comparison and printouts at a later time.

Concerns

1. Limited studies have been done documenting the reliability and validity of information from the system.
2. Manufacturer does not provide accessories to allow isolated movements of all joints.
3. As this equipment has evolved and changes have been made, it has sometimes been difficult to get compatible components. The manufacturer has developed trade-in allowances to allow upgrades if an outmoded system has become problematic.
4. Earlier systems were based on a computer system (Radio Shack) which did not hold up for clinical use (disk drives were also a problem).
5. Service problems are sometimes difficult to address as there are limited technicians for this product.
6. Limited protocols have been developed for this equipment, and it has been difficult to establish user-group activities.
7. Equipment is manufactured by one group but marketed by another and this sometimes leads to difficulties.

Conclusions

Many clinicians feel that this device is a good "exercise" device but has not been developed primarily as a testing tool. The uses of the equipment lend themselves very well to fitness centers but less well to some clinical settings. This is particularly true of the earlier Ariel units with the newer units appearing more flexible and posing promise for evaluative settings. It is imperative that additional clinical studies and reliability/ validity values be established.

Biodex

The Biodex is "user friendly" and enables rapid acquisition of the skills necessary to utilize the equipment. A variety of exercise and testing modes are available to fit a broad patient base. The work hardening accessories allow this unit (along with back accessories) to satisfy nearly all clinical needs. Biodex is a single-product-line company. This is a strength as well as a concern: it implies that all efforts are directed as this product, but it also limits the ability to spread financial liability.

Concerns

1. The accessories (joint, table/chair, etc.) appear at times to be less than "tightly" manufactured; this might lead to early fatigue failure.
2. Problems have been reported with dynamometer heads; these have been promptly replaced through the company replacement policy.
3. Limitation of 150 ft-lb through the eccentric contraction does not allow the assessment of major muscle groups.

Conclusions

The Biodex Corporation has attempted to develop one power head (dynamometer) with a myriad of attachments to perform all forms of testing. Their concept appears to be directed toward enabling a clinic to purchase one unit to accommodate all of its needs. The printouts generated from the system are easily interpreted and provide appropriate information in an easily digested form. This tool appears to be a compromise between high speed (450 degrees/second) and high torque (150 ft-lb, for eccentric contractions). Rather than being able to tolerate high eccentric loads or very high isokinetic speeds, the compromise is to enable the machine to be used for a variety of settings.

Cybex

A primary strength of the Cybex is that it is a known entity. It has been used for a number of years and clinicians are familiar with and comfortable with the information provided by the system. The established service capability and representative system are appreciated by the users. The passive nature of the equipment stresses the safety of the system. The accessories provided enable use for multiple joints with excellent stability of test position. The ability to test manually with computer enhancement is appreciated by many clinicians.

Concerns

1. Because of the passive nature of the system, no eccentrics are available through the Cybex system.
2. Although it is a passive system, velocities cannot exceed 300 degrees/second.
3. Lack of computer storage on the Cybex II and II+ is corrected through the 340 system (we have not yet seen the 340 in clinical use).

Conclusions

The Cybex Company has done an excellent job of bringing isokinetic exercise to the clinical setting. Their educational seminar series is an example of their efforts directed toward this evolution. The concept of computer enhancement has been more fully developed with the introduction of the 340 system. The myriad of attachments designed for the Cybex enable the testing of multiple joints in a reliable fashion. Because the system has been available for a number of years, many research reports are available as well as testing protocols and rehabilitation programs. This makes the Cybex very appealing to large clinics with multiple staff members. Physicians are comfortable with the numbers generated from the Cybex system; this system facilitates communication.

The separate back system is a relatively new area for isokinetic exercise and Cybex has three different devices for specific testing. This area offers great potential but much research is needed.

The safety, reliability, and ease of clinical use make the Cybex an applicable tool for a variety of settings.

Kin-Com

Multiple exercise modes enable individualization of treatment and offer the flexibility of testing a variety of muscle activities. The stability of the system is excellent and the computer control allows storage and collection capabilities. The new computer offers greater independence of use by the clinician and the patient.

The tremendous torque capabilities of the system allow the eccentric testing of most muscle groups. This is particularly important to clinicians involved with research on muscle capabilities of multiple contraction modes.

The distributor, Chattecx, is a subsidiary of Chattanooga. This is viewed as a strong selling point for Kin-Com.

Concerns

1. It is often difficult to simplify the information and thus provide the physician with a clinically oriented report. The newer system provides more clinical data.
2. Some users find specific joint setups are a bit awkward; there is less than adequate stabilization, and the patient does not feel comfortable.
3. The system cannot exceed 210 degrees/second.
4. The system is computer controlled. Although allowing the system to be versatile and adaptable, this presents the problem of not allowing the use of the system if there is a software or a hardware problem.
5. The newest software does not allow the measurement of work power. This may be a concern for clinicians in research settings in which such measurements are becoming increasingly desired.

Conclusions

Many users feel that the Kin-Com is the best device available for settings involving research and clinical applications. They cite the use of electromyography (EMG) and high torque capabilities as being critical to that domain. The company has shown a strong desire to adapt the software to the needs of the users. This enables those centers involved with research to satisfy their needs while allowing the general clinician to have a clinically applicable tool. The evolution of this system has resulted in a more "user friendly" system with enhanced clinical applications. Like the Biodex, the Kin-Com is a compromise between speed and torque. The ability to do high eccentric torques (2200 Newtons) may be such that the unit will not do the higher velocities and thus the 210 degrees/second limitation.

The Kin-Com offers a strong, powerful testing device for a clinical and research environment.

Lido

Comfort is highly praised with this particular system; much of this is attributed to the sliding-cuff. Clinicians have been pleased with the response of the Loredan Company to requests for changes in software applications. The printouts are easily interpreted and present appropriate information. Among the strengths of this system are the visual displays used as a patient motivational tool and the fact that only limited space is required for this instrument.

Concerns

1. The passive Lido system has the limitation of low speed/isometric contractions as well as a lack of eccentrics.
2. The eccentric contraction is based on a concentric contraction and may not allow the testing of eccentric capabilities. Clinicians have indicated they would like to be able to dial in their own limitations rather than base the eccentric contraction on a concentric contraction which may not be reflective of eccentric ability or some pathologic conditions.
3. The multiple safety systems built into the Lido at times have led to problems with the newly introduced active system. I⁺ appears that the safety features may be a bit too sensitive, resulting in the system's being inactivated and requiring technical intervention.

Conclusions

The Lido has evolved from a knee machine into a multijoint evaluation system. The introduction of the back unit further expands the equipment available from this manufacturer. It appears that many patients like the smoothness of the system; this may be related to the sliding-cuff. The reports generated from this system are easily applicable and serve to convey appropriate information quite effectively. The ability to move the equipment rather than the patient also makes this system adaptable to patients with neurologic problems as well as those with orthopedic concerns. Because the active system has only been available recently, we will have to wait to determine how things will evolve.

MERAC

The multiple capabilities of the system include modes of exercise, high velocities, and high torque limitations. Many users feel that this is the most stable exercise system that they have used. Universal is known for its "hardware" and thus this seems appropriate. There are a large number of patterns available and the setups appear to be quite easy, often allowing patient independence.

Concerns

1. Information retrieval is difficult at times and may be facilitated by future development of the software and with greater accessibility of hard drive systems.
2. Users find too much numeric information rather than more simplistic graphic representation on the present printouts. It is almost too much information for easy interpretation.
3. Lack of eccentric capabilities is also a concern.

Conclusions

The MERAC is the newest isokinetic device, and thus it has the least amount of documentation and clinical evaluation. The Universal Company is known for being involved with exercise equipment that is sturdy and functional. Further evaluation in clinical use will determine how well the MERAC performs.

Recommendations

The selection of isokinetic equipment is no longer a simple process. Clinicians should gather as much information as possible on the various devices. Other clinicians have much to share about the most important and applicable features of different kinds of isokinetic equipment. This issue presents basic information that will serve as a starting point.

Different machines will accomplish the task of evaluation in different forms. Thus, it is important to keep in mind that you must not compare apples and oranges. The gravity correction of the different systems will possibly lead to different numbers when comparing the evaluation of a patient using different systems. Do not attempt to compare the torque generated from different devices but rather be aware of the differences and appreciate their importance.

INDEX

Page numbers in *italics* denote figures; those followed by "t" denote tables